Problem-Solving in Nursing Practice

Problem-Solving In Nursing Practice

Keith Hurst, RGN, PhD
Lecturer, Nuffield Institute for Health Services
Studies
University of Leeds

Scutari Press
London

© Scutari Press 1993

A division of Scutari Projects, the publishing company of the Royal College of Nursing

First published 1993

British Library Cataloguing in Publication Data
  Hurst, Keith
  Approaches to Problem Solving in Nursing Practice
  I. Title
  610.73

  ISBN 1-871364-80-9

Typeset by J&L Composition Ltd, Filey, North Yorkshire
Printed and bound in Great Britain by St Edmundsbury Press Ltd
Bury St Edmunds, Suffolk

Contents

Acknowledgements

I am indebted to the following people for their unfailing support during this research:

Dr Stuart Trickey, Ms Anne Dean, Dr Val Reed, Dr John Sheehan, Mr David Brotherhood, Miss Pat McCalman, Mr Ivor Day and colleagues, Mrs Audrey Lathwood and colleagues, Mrs Anne Hill and colleagues, Dr David Thompson, Mr Gerry Bowman, the nurses who validated the vignettes and transcripts, and the informants who kindly agreed to be interviewed.

I am indebted to my wife Jean and daughter Rowan in particular for their patience.

I would also like to thank the Department of Health for their support and guidance.

Preface

One of the requirements for high quality, individualised nursing care is that nurses must recognise and attempt to solve patients' health problems. It is generally agreed that this needs a problem-solving approach.

It was decided to investigate the perceptions and understanding of problem-solving in nursing using a model derived from the general literature. This model, from an analysis of 55 studies, consists of five phases which happen to be similar to the four or five stages in discussions of the nursing process.

Insight into nurses' perceptions of problem-solving was obtained by presenting 120 nurses, in individual interviews, with seven specially constructed and validated vignettes of clinical problem-solving. Deliberately, only one of the vignettes was complete, that is to say, it contained all five elements of the derived model. The other six vignettes had one or more of the elements missing. The nurses were encouraged to comment on each vignette, and the protocols were analysed in detail.

Analysis revealed that the phase model was generally understood by all types of informant, but a number failed to detect the missing phases in some vignettes; in particular, problem identification, planning and evaluation. On the other hand, problem assessment and implementation almost always attracted comment. There did not appear to be a relationship between informants' nursing experience and the recognition or non-recognition of phases. Another finding was that informants were not always systematic in their analysis of the vignettes; that is, some did not begin their analysis with problem identification and conclude with evaluation. Overall, the findings lend support to a stages model as a theoretical basis for problem-solving in nursing.

The theoretical basis of problem-solving in nursing is also discussed in relation to problem-solving in allied professional disciplines. Finally, the implications of the study for nursing education and practice are explained and recommendations made for further study.

This development of a problem-solving approach to nursing has been one of the more important changes that has taken place in nursing during the 1980s. There has been a significant shift from nursing's traditional disease-oriented approach to care, to a patient-centred, problem-solving approach (Beswetherick, 1979; Henderson, 1982). Traditional nursing is dominated by the medical model, that is, the patient's nursing care is directed by doctors' orders (Clarke, 1978; Boylan, 1982). Traditional practitioners see the patient as a repository of disease, with the main goal being to alleviate symptoms. Consequently, the curriculum for this type of nursing included the didactic transmission of general nursing principles, coupled with the imparting of recipes of specific nursing care to be used according to the patient's disease or symptoms (Boylan, 1982; Hardy and Engel, 1987).

Critics of traditional nursing felt that nurses were merely handmaidens to doctors and lacked autonomy. Because of its task-centred nature and its use of rigid nursing procedures, it is argued that traditional nursing fails to make full use of the nurse's problem-solving skills (de la Cuesta, 1983; Kershaw, 1987). As a result of this concern, some nurses rejected traditional nursing in favour of a patient-centred model of care (Docking and Neave, 1986).

1

Introduction

The development of a problem-solving approach in nursing

Nurses today have to be more skilled in problem-solving than ever before. Changes in their professional role have meant that they are often in novel situations for which their previous experience has not prepared them, and a personal, all-encompassing problem-solving strategy has to be employed. Nurses have more contact with patients than any other professional group and thus have the greatest opportunity to apply their knowledge to meet the patients' needs.

Early attempts to develop patient-centred care employed patient-allocated nursing. In this situation, a team of nurses provides the total care for a small group of patients. Because the work is coordinated by a team leader, the nurse's problem-solving skills are still under-utilised (Beswetherick, 1979; Kershaw, 1987). However, further developments have led to the introduction of individualised nursing care, an approach in which the nurse plans, delivers and evaluates the care of one patient, based on the assessment of that patient. Nurse practitioners and educators realised that individualised nursing care depended on intellectual as well as practical nursing skills (Yura and Walsh, 1978, p. 93; Basford et al., 1987). To meet these concerns, the use of a problem-solving approach in nurse education and practice was encouraged by the General Nursing Council (1977).

Nurses have, in recent years, concentrated on the provision of individualised care. In so doing British nurses have paid considerable attention to nursing developments in North America, in particular, the nursing process and nursing models (Aggleton and Chalmers, 1986). The nursing process, one systematic method of delivering individualised nursing care, consists of, in turn, patient assessment, identification of nursing problems, application of nursing care to solve these problems and evaluation of outcome (Yura and Walsh, 1978, Chapter 3).

Nursing models, of which there are several variants, are supportive to and supported by the nursing process. Models of nursing enhance the systematic and cohesive nature of the nursing process (Aggleton and Chalmers, 1984). The nursing process, in conjunction with nursing models, provides a framework for nursing, helping nurses to organise their work and develop nursing knowledge and practice (Henderson, 1982). Both models and process rely on the nurse's problem-solving skills (Aggleton and Chalmers, 1984).

It must be stressed, however, that although the nursing process is a popular approach to individualised patient care (de la Cuesta, 1983), it is only one approach to problem-solving in nursing. In fact, there is no consensus model of clinical problem-solving. There are relatively few practical and theoretical studies in this area and empirical evidence is slender. Relevant studies will be discussed in Chapter 3.

It is contended that problem-solving is an important but poorly understood feature of modern nursing. A sound understanding of this process is a major requirement of high-quality patient care and the development of professional skills (see e.g. Wooley et al., 1974; Bailey and Claus, 1975; Corcoran, 1986; UKCC, 1987; Tanner et al., 1987). It is hoped that this research will increase understanding of this process through the study of nurses' perceptions of problem-solving in clinical settings.

Definition of terms

Before an attempt is made to describe the theories of problem-solving, we shall define the concepts central to this study. This section is divided into two parts: the first covers definitions of problem-solving in general contexts, and the second defines problem-solving in nursing.

Problem-solving in general

The definition of problem-solving

The definition of problem-solving is dependent on the definition of problem and solution. A problem is said to exist either when there is a discrepancy between the actual and the ideal state of affairs, or when an individual cannot immediately assimilate a situation and cannot satisfy a need (see e.g. Schmuck et al., 1966, p. 15; Newell and Simon, 1972, pp. 72–3; Bailey and Claus, 1975, p. 20; Simon and Hayes, 1985, p. 253). The former definition is usually applied to well-defined problems. An ill-defined problem, on the other hand, is said to be a situation where there is no apparent relationship between certain initial information and the goal (see e.g. Merrifield et al., 1962, p. 1; Chi and Glaser, 1984, p. 246; Kahney, 1986, p. 15). A solution is usually defined as the achievement of a specified goal, following a series of actions to reach the goal (Wickelgren, 1973, p. 16).

Although definitions of problem-solving include common features, they tend to be context-dependent (Hill, 1979, pp. 15–16; Munro, 1982, p. 46). That is, the interpretation of problem-solving by an educationalist includes educational descriptors in the definition (Schmuck et al., 1966, p. 15), and that of a manager includes management concepts (Margerison, 1974, pp. 24–8). For example, Huckabay (1980, p. 126) gives a detailed definition specific to education:

> The process of problem solving may be viewed as a form of principle learning in which the learner discovers a combination of previously learned lower-level rules and applies them in the learning of higher-order rules, thus achieving a solution for a novel problem situation.

Cox and Ewan (1982, pp. 11–13) agree with Huckabay on the importance of 'principle learning' and include it in their description. Bloom et al. (1956, p. 38) highlight the significance of novelty and higher-order thinking in their explanation of problem-solving. De Tornyay (1970, p. 85) summarises these key features:

> Problem solving, an extremely important objective in learning, consists of discovery because the learner is expected to generate a novel combination of previously learned principles. It is a synthesising of understanding towards a solution.

Tuckman (1978, p. 359), an educational psychologist, sees problem-solving as the ability to identify and describe solutions to problem situations that have not been encountered before and cannot be produced through memory. Gagné (1966, pp. 129–32), on the other hand, believes that successful problem-solving depends on the solver's ability to recall knowledge of related facts and concepts.

Clearly, problem-solving in general situations is more than just the recall of a solution; it involves a synthesis of new information derived from existing knowledge. Successful problem-solving also seems to depend on several cognitive abilities, including lower- and higher-order thinking – for example, the learning of simple and complex rules. These definitions of problem-solving can be compared with those specific to nursing.

Problem-solving in nursing contexts

Abdellah's (1957, p. 6) definition of a nursing problem is based on nurse–patient interaction, and is therefore context-tied. According to her a nursing problem is 'a condition and/or situation faced by a patient, or his family, which the nurse can assist him to meet through the performance of her professional function'. Ashworth and Castledine's (1981, p. 88) more detailed definition of a nursing problem also recognises the nurse–patient relationship. They state:

> A nursing problem can be defined as any condition or situation in which a patient requires nursing assistance or help to attain, maintain or regain, a state of health which is desirable for him, or to achieve a peaceful death . . .

The nurse–patient interaction is implicit within many definitions of problem-solving in nursing. Some definitions also describe a systematic process, consisting of well-defined steps (Wenk, 1981, p. 216). For example, Johnson et al. (1980, pp. 1–2) state that problem-solving 'consists of a series of definite steps which proceed in a logical manner toward a specific goal. These steps are: assessment, development of a plan, implementation of the plan and evaluation.'

Some nurses also stress its cyclical nature, that is, evaluation is usually followed by a return to one of the preceding steps (Yura and Walsh, 1978, pp. 91–3).

The similarity between Yura and Walsh's definition of the nursing process and Johnson et al.'s is very clear. In fact, nursing process and nursing problem-solving are concepts that tend to be used synonymously in the literature (Henderson, 1982). However, in this study, the terms 'nursing process' and 'problem-solving' are assigned separate meanings because the nursing process is considered to be only one method of solving nursing problems. Also, the nursing process is only applicable to patient care, whereas problem-solving can be applied to clinical, managerial and educational contexts.

2

Theories of Problem-solving

The literature on problem-solving is vast, and covers many disciplines and perspectives. An inspection of the early literature on problem-solving reveals approaches that relate to contemporary psychological theories. These include the Gestalt theory of problem-solving (Forehand, 1966, p. 356), the psychometric theory (Forehand, 1966, p. 357) and the behavioural theory (Skinner, 1966, pp. 225–58). More recent approaches fall into two broad categories: the information-processing system theory (Newell and Simon, 1972, pp. 787–868) and the stages model theory of problem-solving, of which there are many variants (Hill, 1979, p. 16).

The information-processing system theory

Newell and Simon introduced this new and highly influential theory of problem-solving in the 1960s and published their major research in 1972 (Newell and Simon, 1972). This seminal work has been developed and refined in recent years by Simon and Hayes (1985, Chapter 12), as well as by other writers (see e.g. Chi and Glaser, 1984, Chapter 10; Kahney, 1986, pp. 39–49).

The theory postulates that problem-solving is a product of elementary information-processing activities, which form a framework of three interlinked components: (1) task environment; (2) problem space; and (3) problem-solving strategy (Simon and Hayes, 1985, pp. 254–61).

When faced with a problem, and depending on its complexity, the solver may quickly realise the solution or decide that a solution is attainable by selecting a strategy to solve the problem (Newell and Simon, 1972, pp. 787–90).

First, as Chi and Glaser (1984, pp. 232–3) and Kahney (1986, pp. 39–41) explain, there is an understanding process, which helps the solver to formulate a problem space (the problem-solver's representation of the problem) from the task environment (the external representation of the problem). The formulation of the problem space is the point where the solver activates part of his or her rich knowledge base, selecting elements which are felt to be essential to understanding the problem and to developing the solution (Simon and Hayes, 1985, pp. 258–61; Kahney, 1986, p. 40). The problem space is, therefore, an important part of problem-solving because it contains all the relevant information, including the solution.

The problem-solver may alternate between the 'understanding process' and the third element of the information-processing system, the problem-solving strategy. This helps the solver to interpret the problem further and construct a problem-solving strategy through an exploration of the problem space (Chi and Glaser, 1984, p. 234). Searching the problem space is primarily a move from one node (a chunk of related information) to another (Simon and Hayes, 1985, p. 260), and one (or a combination) of the following strategies may be used:

1. random searching (indiscriminate searching for goals);
2. heuristic search (using rules of thumb);
3. means–ends analysis (reducing discrepancy between actual and ideal state);
4. sub-goaling (breaking down the problem into intermediate states);
5. generation and testing (of possible solutions).

(Chi and Glaser, 1984, pp. 234–9; Kahney, 1986, pp. 39–46). For example, the solver may break the problem down into sub-problems and identify goals by drawing in new information from the task environment. Another strategy could begin with (1) goal selection; (2) working towards the goal by applying operators; and (3) ending with evaluation. These actions help to generate solutions (Newell and Simon, 1972, Chapter 14).

Information-processing is a dynamic process, that is, the solver may compare new experiences with past ones and may store the products for short- and long-term use. The solver may also employ an external memory (for example, written notes), particularly when large amounts of information are being manipulated (Newell and Simon, 1972, pp. 788–803; Wickelgren, 1973, pp. 91–3; Simon and Hayes, 1985, pp. 260–4; Kahney, 1986, pp. 137–40).

Information-processing theorists feel that people differ in the way they solve problems for a number of reasons (Simon and Hayes, 1985, p. 266). For example, individuals employ different strategies because of the different ways the problem has been perceived and because of the different amounts of knowledge and experience held (Newell and Simon, 1972, pp. 787–9; Kahney, 1986, p. 41). This variation can be seen when comparing the problem-solving behaviour of novices and experts (Kahney, 1986, pp. 102–7). Experience, however, is no guarantee that the problem will be solved (Newell and Simon, 1972, pp. 847–52).

Many supporters of the information-processing system theory believe it to be the most promising way of examining and describing the complex behaviour of problem-solving. It is evident that the theory encourages the detailed study and description of the cognitive processes of problem-solving in contrast to the more general approach of the stages model theory (and other theories) (Green, 1966, pp. 3–16).

Our knowledge of the information-processing theory is incomplete, however (Simon and Hayes, 1985, p. 266). The theory appears to be particularly weak in its explanation of solving ill-defined problems. The application of the theory to more complex problems, such as real-life ones, seems to have been less successful (Chi and Glaser, 1984, p. 239), perhaps because the bulk of the research has been conducted under laboratory conditions using well-defined (puzzle) problems (Chi and Glaser, 1984, p. 246; Simon and Hayes, 1985, p. 253).

Stages model theory

The second major approach to describing the problem-solving process is the stage, or step-wise, model of problem-solving (Green, 1966, p. 11; Hill, 1979, p. 16). The number of accounts explaining the process of problem-solving in this way is extensive (Johnson, 1944; Hill, 1979, p. 16). One list, displaying 55 different representations of stages models gathered from a major review of the general and specific literature on problem-solving spanning the past 50 years, is summarised in Table 2.1. The number of stages in each separate model varies considerably, ranging from three (Johnson, 1944) to ten (Bailey and Claus, 1975, Chapter 3). There are many similarities in the names used and the processes identified (Priestley et al., 1979, pp. 99–101).

This complex picture is simplified by Priestley et al., who explain:

> In essence they are simply formulae that guide us into activities – things to do that will make solutions to problems more readily available . . . they cannot guarantee answers: they do lead us by a series of logical steps to conclusions that are unique and inviolable. For the most part they produce ideas in quantity, for which a solution can be chosen . . . (ibid., pp. 100–1)

This statement, and the authors' discussion, indicate the systematic and pragmatic nature of the stages model theory. It has wide application, ranging from everyday problems of living, to situations which may involve complex human problem-solving. There is, however, a difficulty of manageability with the many descriptions of problem-solving. A citation count of the named, individual stages cited in Table 2.1 is given in Table 2.2.

We can see that there is considerable overlap between one stage and the next; for example, 'selection and implementation of strategies' (2), and 'planning interventions' (4) could be combined into one. Combining stages

Table 2.1 Stages models of problem-solving citing the author's naming and sequence of stages

Key to stages

(PId) Problem identification/orienting
(PDe) Problem definition
(PAn) Problem/sub-problem analysis
(PAs) Problem assessment/data collection
(Go) Goal/objective setting
(Hy) Hypothesis formation/testing
(Di) Diagnosing
(Pr) Preparation
(PIn) Planning interventions
(Im) Selection/implementation of strategies
(Ge) Generation/production of solutions
(T) Testing
(L) Learning
(Ev) Evaluation/verification of solution
(Re) Re-appraisal of problem
(G) Generalisation

Author (Only first author cited)		Stages															
		PId	PDe	PAn	PAs	Go	Di	Hy	PIn	Pr	Im	Ge	T	L	Ev	Re	G
Wallas	(1926)	1		2								3			4		
Chrisof	(1939)	1			2				2		3				3		
Johnson	(1944)	1			2				2			2			3		
Johnson	(1955)									1		2			3		
Dawson	(1956)	1		2								3			4		5
Thomson	(1959)	1	1	3	2				3		4	4					
Merrifield	(1962)	1		2	2							3			4	5	
Polya	(1963)	1		2	2				3		4				4		
Gagné	(1966)	1	2					3							4		
Green	(1966)	1		2								3					
Kron	(1966)	1	1		2						4	3			5		
Schmuck	(1966)	1					2		3		4				5		
Shone	(1974)			3	2	1			4		5						
Bailey	(1975)	1	2	3		5			4&6		7&9	6			8&10		
Johnson	(1975)				1&4		2		5		3&5						
Walter	(1976)		1		1	2			3						4		
Boreham	(1977)	2			1				3		4						
Feightner	(1977)	1			2			3									
Elstein	(1978)			2	1			3							4		
Sculco	(1978)	1		2					3		3				4		
Vitale	(1978)			2	1		3	4			5				6		
Yura	(1978)				1				2		3				4		
Hill	(1979)				1				2		3					4	
Priestley	(1979)				1	2								3	4		
Vu	(1979)				1			2			4				3		
Yeaw	(1979)	1							2			3	4				
Crow	(1980)				1				2		3				4		
Darcy	(1980)				1		2		3		4				5		
Huckabay	(1980)	1	2					3							4		
Johnson	(1980)			2	1				3		4				5		
Teare	(1980)		1			1			2		3			5	4		
Ashworth	(1981)				1				2		3				4		
Goble	(1981)	1	2			1			6		6	3&5			4		
Joorabchi	(1981)	1		4	3			2&6	5				7				
McCarthy	(1981)				1				2		3				4		
Egan	(1982)		2	3	1	4			5		6&7				8		
Henderson	(1982)	1			1				2		3				4		
Kaufman	(1982)	1			1	2			2		3				4		
Greenwood	(1983)	1		2	1	3					4				5		

Table 2.1 Continued.

King	(1983)	1				2				3		4		5	
Richardson	(1984)	1			3	2						4			
Sugden	(1984)	1				1				2		3		4	
Hollingworth	(1985)					1				2		3		4	
Jones	(1985)	1	2							4		5	3	6	
Phillips	(1985)	1	1	1				2		3					
Sheaf	(1985)	1	1	1	2					2		3		3	3
Breckman	(1986)	1	1	1	2					3		3		4	
Brightman	(1986)						2		1	4	3				
Cousins	(1986)					1				2		3		4	
Beeler	(1987)	1				2				4			3	5	
Greaves	(1987)	1	2			3				2		5		4&6	
Harris	(1987)	1					2					3		4	
HCEA	(1987)	1	2							5		5	3	4&6	
Pardue	(1987)					1		2		3		4		5	
Marriner-Tomey	(1988)	1	2	3						4		5		6	

Table 2.2 A citation count of the stages in Table 2.1

Rank Order	Stages	Number of citations
1.	Evaluation/verification of solution	47
2.	Selection and implementation of strategies	44
3.	Problem assessment and data collection	40
4.	Planning interventions	38
5.	Problem identification	34
6.	Problem/sub-problem analysis	23
7.	Generation of solutions	15
8.	Goal/objective setting	11
9.	Hypothesis formation	10
10.	Problem definition	10
11.	Diagnosis	6
12.	Re-appraisal of problem	3
13.	Teaching	3
14.	Preparation	2
15.	Learning	2
16.	Generalisation	1

of a similar name is one way of condensing the sixteen elements. Alternatively, the list of stages can be made more manageable by taking the five most frequently cited stages and calculating the mean placing of each. For example, in Table 2.1, 'problem identification' (PId) is cited 34 times. The mean placing of this stage is 1, that is, it is consistently cited as the first step in problem-solving. The result of applying a similar procedure to the other four most common stages is given in Table 2.3.

Table 2.3 The mean place of the five most frequently cited stages from Table 2.2

Sequence	Stage	Mean place
1.	Problem identification	1.0
2.	Problem assessment/data collection	1.5
3.	Planning interventions	3.0
4.	Selection and implementation of strategies	4.0
5.	Evaluation/verification of solution	4.4

Table 2.4 The main problem-solving stages used in this research

Stages* used in this research	Corresponding 'stages' from Table 2.1	Key
1. Problem identification		
	(a) problem identification	(PId)
	(b) problem definition	(PDe)
2. Problem assessment		
	(a) problem/sub-problem analysis	(PAn)
	(b) problem assess./data collection	(PAs)
3. Planning interventions		
	(a) goal/objective setting	(Go)
	(b) hypothesis formation	(Hy)
	(c) planning interventions	(PIn)
	(d) generating solutions	(Ge)
4. Implementation		
	(a) selecting/implementing strategies	(Im)
5. Evaluation		
	(a) evaluation/verification	(Ev)
	(b) re-appraisal of problem	(Re)

* Later in this book these are referred to as 'phases' rather than stages (this is explained more fully in Chapter 5, p. 47).

In summarising and simplifying the extensive literature on stages models of problem-solving in this way, we arrive at a five-stage model, which can be applied to research in many disciplines. The stages model used in this research has as its basis this five-stage model. Each stage can be further qualified (Table 2.4).

There are some finer points in the explanations of stages models which are worthy of note. Considerable emphasis is placed on the sequential and cyclical nature of the model (Gagné, 1966, pp. 129–48; Sculco, 1978; Johnson et al., 1980, pp. 5–7; Jones and Sado, 1985). Indeed, these characteristics are evident in many of the stages models identified in Table 2.1.

Further, the problem-solver, depending on the difficulty of the problem and his or her experience, can enter the model at any stage, but usually begins with problem identification, and progresses through the other stages in a linear fashion (Bailey and Claus, 1975, pp. 10–18; Joorabchi, 1981).

In fact, those studies that have examined successful and unsuccessful problem-solving indicate that subjects who approach the problem in a systematic, selective and reflective way tend to be successful (Attree, 1982, pp. 2–7). As Yeaw (1979, p. 18) explains: 'The successful problem-solvers were more systematic. They divided the problems and simplified the facts. Students who were less successful tended to "dive in" attempting to solve the whole problem.'

Successful problem-solving requires a number of skills, according to the problem situation. Generally, these can be grouped under the headings 'intellectual' and 'practical' skills (see Bloom et al., 1956, p. 103; Bailey and Claus, 1975, pp. 18–28; Woditsch, 1978, pp. 236–57; Priestley et al., 1979, Chapter 5; Yeaw, 1979; Callin and Ciliska, 1983; Woodbury, 1984; Hollingworth, 1985, p. 44).

The stages model theory has several strengths, of which the most important, arguably, is that the step-by-step method of identifying and solving problems encourages systematic thinking habits, which can be transferred to other problem contexts (Priestley et al., 1979, pp. 99–101). A second strength is that in the case of unsuccessful problem-solving, it is possible to isolate the weak link or links and implement remedial action (Bailey and Claus, 1975, p. 110). Third, the model demonstrates flexibility, both in its application to different problem situations and in the partial use of stages according to the complexity of the problem (Johnson et al., 1980, Chapter 1). Fourth, stages models are used to teach and facilitate learning (Hill, 1979, pp. 85–100) as well as explain the process of problem-solving (ibid., pp. 18–21).

Perhaps the greatest difference between the information-processing system and the stages model theories of problem-solving is the context and type of problem studied. The information-processing theorists have focused their research on well-defined, puzzle-like problems in laboratory settings. The stages model theory, on the other hand, tends to be applied to both well-defined and complex real-life problems (Priestley et al., 1979, p. 99).

The stages model theory is, however, open to criticism because much of the literature has no empirical base. Some stages model theorists recommend strategies for solving problems that are not supported by research, whereas in the case of the information-processing theory, interpretations are generally well supported by evidence. Information-processing theorists have tried to demonstrate that problem-solving is more than a chaining together of discrete, rigidly bound stages, where every event can be isolated from the others. Moreover, it is argued that some of the processes are carried out rapidly with the blurring of one stage into another, and includes thought processes which occur concurrently (Green, 1966, p. 12).

Other critics have pointed out that not all the stages can be fitted into a universal problem-solving model and that some models contain inappropriate stages (Forehand, 1966, pp. 361–4; Hill, 1979, p. 16). For example, Priestley et al. (1979, p. 71) include 'learning' as a separate stage in their model (see Table 2.1). Arguably, 'learning' is part of all problem-solving stages and the authors' reasoning that 'learning' is a distinct stage is unconvincing.

There is also concern that one or more stages in the process can be omitted and yet a solution can still be obtained (Forehand, 1966, pp. 361–4; Hill, 1979, p. 16). It is for these reasons that the stages model theory is seen by some as an inadequate explanation of problem-solving behaviour see Forehand, 1966, pp. 362–3; Green, 1966, pp. 11–12; Newell and Simon, 1972, p. 869).

In addition, nurses who concentrate on stages models may be ignoring the rapidly growing body of knowledge from research into diagnostic reasoning in nursing in which problem-solving is used to determine a patient's nursing needs (Carnevali et al., 1984, pp. 40–41). This research, based on the information-processing theory, has demonstrated sub-processes of problem-solving that appear more complex than some stages models in total (Carnevali et al., 1984, pp. 25–53; Tanner, 1986). These issues will be examined in more detail in Chapter 3.

In summary, the stages model theory of problem-solving, with the reservations mentioned above, describes the problem-solving process in a clear, logical and manageable way. It also provides a framework for the study, teaching and practice of problem-solving. The theory is flexible; and the whole or part of it can be applied to all problems. Examples of these applications will be discussed in the next two chapters.

3

Problem-solving in Nursing

The literature on problem-solving in nursing falls broadly into two categories; the information-processing system and the stages model theories. But there is, lamentably, little empirical evidence regarding the actual problem-solving strategies used by nurses. Some authors, writing generally, tend to discuss problem-solving in an anecdotal way and suggest how problem-solving ought to be done rather than how it is done. Another difficulty is that much of the work in this area has been carried out in North America and needs to be tested in UK nursing contexts before it can be applied to nursing here. This work is examined later. Authors who use the information-processing system theory to explain clinical problem-solving include Yura and Walsh (1978, Chapter 2), McCarthy (1981) and Tanner et al. (1987). Following the procedure in the previous chapter, this theory is examined first.

Information-processing system theory in relation to nursing

As we saw in Chapter 2 (pp. 5–7), the information-processing system theory has three components: (1) task environment; (2) problem space; and (3) problem-solving strategy. Yura and Walsh (1978, pp. 55–65) discuss the information-processing system theory in much the same way as writers in the general literature, and feel that the information-processing theory is particularly helpful in explaining the act of nursing problem-solving.

They suggest (ibid., pp. 55–6) that the task environment, from which a nurse formulates the problem space, determines the nature of the problem-solving endeavour. They also explain that the problem space is not a real space but the nurse's mental picture, which is based on an understanding of the problem, the nurse's immediate thought processes when meeting the problem, and his or her knowledge of and experience with similar situations. The problem space also includes the goals, rules and procedures, and any other concepts seen to be appropriate to the problem and solution.

It is felt that an accurate and complete problem space is crucial to successful problem-solving; it helps the nurse to organise the problem-solving strategy, which is mainly a search for the solution by identifying, analysing and synthesising knowledge within the problem space (ibid., pp. 55–6).

Yura and Walsh go on to describe a variety of problem-solving strategies which may be used by the nurse. For example, the experienced problem-solver sometimes recognises the solution to the problem simply by recalling a similar problem. However, as we have seen from the definitions in Chapter 1 (p. 2), problem-solving is more than just recall.

Trial-and-error is a problem-solving strategy in which potential solutions are implemented until a successful outcome is achieved. At other times a more sustained search may be required before a solution is reached. For example, hypothesis-generation and testing is a strategy in which possible solutions are generated to guide the search for information to confirm a solution. Evaluation of progress towards a solution also features as a problem-solving strategy. This type of evaluation may be formative or summative, and provides feedback for the problem-solver. In other situations, however, it may become clear to the nurse that a solution to a difficult problem is unattainable.

During the search for a solution, the nurse may recognise new problems, which may need to take priority or be set aside for later work. Because of the influx of new information from the problem environment, new goals may be established. It is for these reasons that a nurse's clinical problem-solving is sometimes linear, sometimes branching and other times cyclical.

There are many factors which determine the nurse's choice of a problem-solving strategy. He or she may consider the potential solution with regard to the safety and comfort of the patient, or efficiency and convenience for the carers. The short- and long-term implications for both patient and nurse also need to be considered, so that the best possible solution strategy is chosen and implemented (Yura and Walsh, 1978, pp. 62–3).

The amount of learning which takes place in problem-solving is emphasised by both Yura and Walsh (1978, pp. 56–7) and Kahney (1986, pp. 39–46). It is said that the products of problem-solving are stored in both short-term memory for immediate use and in long-term memory for both immediate and future use. Novice and expert problem-solvers demonstrate different uses of short- and long-term memory, and this may explain the alleged different problem-solving styles of a learner nurse and a ward sister (McCarthy, 1981). As we shall see later in this chapter, these issues are important in one form of problem-solving known as diagnostic reasoning.

The information-processing system theory has, however, been criticised when used in a nursing context. McCarthy (1981) suggests that the ways nurses solve problems are so diverse that this theory is far too limited as an explanation of the process. On the other hand, the literature explaining nursing problem-solving in this way can at best be described as meagre and such criticisms may be unjustified because, as yet, so little is known about the application of the theory to nursing. One reason for the dearth of research is that, as we have seen in Chapter 2 (p. 5), the information-processing system theory of problem-solving is strongly associated with well-defined problems, such as puzzle-like problems (Simon and Hayes, 1985, p. 253). There is very little application, particularly in the United Kingdom, to real life and less well-structured problems, such as those found in nursing.

Diagnostic reasoning

In a rapidly expanding area of study, North American researchers have applied the information-processing system theory and associated research methods to help their understanding of diagnostic reasoning (Carnevali et al., 1984, Chapter 2; Westfall et al., 1986; Tanner et al., 1987). One of the reasons for the growth of this work was the researchers' dissatisfaction with traditional explanations of nursing problem-solving, which are felt to hamper clinical reasoning because of the formalised thinking process. The nursing process is one example of what Carnevali et al. (1984, p. 46) and Tanner et al. (1987) call traditional approaches, since it is a linear method of problem-solving (Hardy and Engel, 1987).

Diagnostic reasoning is defined as a process of determining the patient's health needs using diagnostic hypotheses (Itano, 1989). Carnevali et al. (1984, pp. 40–2) and Jones (1988) emphasise that the term 'diagnosis' in nursing is not used in the narrow sense of identifying disease, but rather to describe the process which leads to conclusions derived from assessment of the patient's health and related factors. Once the nursing diagnosis is made, the nurse then implements nursing actions to mitigate the patient's problem (Yura and Walsh, 1978, pp. 59–60; Tanner et al., 1987). Jones (1988) believes that nursing diagnoses help foster professional autonomy and accountability because their use emphasises the nurse's unique function.

Tanner et al. (1987) feel that the methods and results of diagnostic reasoning research are both interesting and important, and have been a particularly fruitful way of describing the way nurses arrive at a nursing diagnosis. In practice, researchers have tended to compare the cognitive processes of expert and novice nurses by studying qualified and learner nurses' mental reasoning when faced with a simulated patient's problems. Subjects are asked to think aloud from the time they first encounter the patient until a satisfactory nursing diagnosis is established.

The findings suggest that both expert and novice nurses establish early tentative diagnoses when solving clinical problems. It is felt that diagnoses help reduce the cognitive strain associated with remembering large quantities of information and hence their early showing in the problem encounter. Initial diagnoses are weak because of incomplete data, so the nurse searches for evidence to strengthen, modify or reject hypotheses (Tanner et al., 1987; Jones, 1988; Itano, 1989).

Findings also show that experts differ from novices in their data-gathering techniques. Experts are more systematic and better able to recognise important cues. Their final diagnosis tends to be more accurate because of their greater experience. In short, experts are better able to (1) select relevant information; (2) recognise patterns in the data; and (3) manage information (Carnevali et al., 1984, p. 40; Tanner et al., 1987; Jones, 1988; Itano, 1989).

Research into diagnostic reasoning has attracted criticism, not least because studies have tended to be conducted in non-clinical situations. That is, nurses, usually subjects in a sample of convenience, are tested using written, audio or video media describing patients and their problems. The testing situation is particularly important in diagnostic reasoning research because context may be a confounding variable. This may explain why there have been conflicting findings from research which has compared novice and expert diagnostic reasoning in different settings (Pardue, 1987; Tanner et al., 1987). Tanner et al. (1987) and Itano (1989) feel that problem-solving research findings are sensitive to both the task and the context in which the research is carried out.

The researcher feels that workers examining diagnostic reasoning must also be criticised for their limited view of problem-solving. Diagnostic reasoning implies that once the nursing diagnosis has been confirmed, the problem has been solved. In fact, problem-solving has to start afresh from this point to determine the most appropriate nursing interventions. In short, diagnostic reasoning is more closely associated with the finer points of understanding and labelling the problem rather than solving it (McGuire, 1985; Westfall et al., 1986). This may also explain why the literature on information-processing and diagnostic reasoning is con-siderable, but the related literature on planning and evaluating nursing interventions is minimal although no less important (Carnevali et al., 1984, pp. 25–50; Tanner et al., 1987).

Diagnostic reasoning is arguably a valid problem-solving strategy in North American contexts because nursing diagnoses feature strongly in nursing care (Tanner et al., 1987). But nursing diagnosis is a new concept in the United Kingdom. Here, nurses have tended to focus on the patient's problems and needs within the nursing plan, rather than on the formula-tion of nursing diagnoses (McCarthy, 1981; Roper et al., 1983, p. 13). Therefore, the diagnostic reasoning strategy may need fresh thinking in order for it to be seen as appropriate to nursing in the United Kingdom. This does not mean that diagnostic reasoning is ignored by UK nurses.

A review of the UK literature has revealed some important work, albeit not empirical. For example, both Marks-Maran (1983) and Draper (1986) provide reasoned arguments for the substitution of nursing problem with nursing diagnosis in the nursing process. Also, Jones (1988) discusses the teaching and practice of diagnostic reasoning as a means of solving nursing problems, and Sharples (1987) examines diagnoses from a managerial perspective in explaining the importance of medical and nursing diagnosis in the development of the Resource Management Initiative.

It is suggested in this literature that the introduction of nursing diagnosis would be unpopular and may even be resisted by UK nurses. The authors feel, however, that the introduction of nursing diagnosis would be an important if not inevitable step in nursing.

In summary, nursing problem-solving has been interpreted within the framework of the information-processing system theory. But the interpretation is incomplete because of a lack of empirical work, particularly in the United Kingdom. There is a clear need to test this theory in relation to planning, implementing and evaluating the patient's nursing care (McCarthy, 1981; Carnevali et al., 1984, pp. 237–8; Holzemer, 1986).

Literature on the stages model theory of problem-solving in nursing is examined next, though again, empirical work is meagre.

The stages model theory of problem-solving in nursing

Most accounts of nursing problem-solving tend to involve the use of the stages model theory of problem-solving (see Bailey and Claus, 1975; Vitale et al., 1978; Yura and Walsh, 1978; Johnson et al., 1980). One possible explanation for this emphasis is that nursing models and nursing process both have a structure similar to stages models of problem-solving. As discussed in Chapter 1 (pp. 1–2), nursing models and the nursing process are used to support descriptions of modern nursing practice.

The nursing process and nursing models have provided much of the direction for nursing practice in recent years (see pp. 1–2). This is principally because the nursing process, supported by an appropriate model, is a common nursing approach for individualised care and one method of solving a patient's problems (Johnson et al., 1980, pp. 1–11). Another reason for its popularity is that it helps the nurse to clarify and justify nursing an an independent discipline (McCarthy, 1981). According to Vitale et al. (1978, p. 87):

> Nurses are presently working in a variety of settings and are caring for patients with a multiplicity of needs . . . . The problem solving process assists the nurses in caring for patients' complex needs. It is a process that can be utilized in all settings of nursing practice. A process that enables the nurse to scientifically identify a patient's nursing needs and to plan,

implement, and evaluate care through the use of critical thinking is the problem solving process.

Some authors consider the nursing process to be synonymous with problem-solving, for example, Henderson (1982, p. 109):

> Use of the term nursing process, as I have known it, is traced from the 1950s, when I heard it discussed as a way of describing client–nurse communication . . . until the present when it is used to mean problem solving by the nurse for the benefit of the patient.

The steps in the nursing process are set out in Table 3.1 alongside the stages model given in Table 2.4.

It is clear that the two models compare favourably. The major difference is that in the nursing process the identification of the problem is implicit within the assessment stage. Otherwise, the four basic stages are very similar. Since the five stages of the stages model theory are fundamental to modern nursing, each will be described in detail.

1. Problem identification

As we have seen (p. 3), a nursing problem is a disturbance or a potential disturbance in a patient's health state, which requires a nurse's intervention. The first and one of the most important steps in the stages model of clinical problem-solving is an initial gathering and analysing of data followed by problem identification (Vitale et al., 1978, p. 59). This is borne out by the data in Table 2.2, which show that problem identification appears in 34 of the 55 stages models presented in Table 2.1. In some stages models, however, problem identification bears a different name: for example, in Table 2.1 Walter et al. (1976) use the term 'problem definition'. In many stage models, problem identification is subsumed under 'problem assessment' (e.g. Johnson et al., 1975; Pardue, 1987). Interestingly, it is generally nursing writers who do this and whose thinking may have been influenced by the nursing process.

More specifically, problem identification is achieved by interviewing and

Table 3.1 The stages model of problem solving in relation to the nursing process

Stages from the literature	Steps in the nursing process
1. Problem identification	1. Assessment
2. Problem assessment	2. Planning
3. Planning interventions	3. Implementation
4. Implementation	4. Evaluation
5. Evaluation	(Bloch, 1974, p. 689)

selective observation of the patient (Bailey and Claus, 1975, p. 48; Johnson et al., 1980, pp. 56–7). In some cases the patient may pinpoint the problem. At other times, someone else – the patient's relative or doctor, for example – may indicate a problem (Johnson et al., 1980, pp. 47–54; Roper et al., 1983, p. 10; Buckenham, 1986).

A nurse faced with a patient manifesting several problems may classify them in various ways. One way is to label them as actual or potential problems (Roper et al., 1983, p. 10); another is to classify them according to their biological, psychological and social effect (Kron, 1966, p. 136). At other times it may be necessary to prioritise them (Bailey and Claus, 1975, pp. 40–1). Whichever classification is used, Barnett (1985) suggests that the nurse should state the problem in a clear and unambiguous way.

It is claimed that experienced nurses are more able than junior colleagues to formulate a patient's nursing problems. This suggests that problem formulation depends on the nurse's knowledge, experience and clinical judgement (Vitale et al., 1978, p. 63; Corcoran, 1986). Skeet and Thompson (1985) studied learner nurses' performance on their final examination. The researchers demonstrated that the learner's failure to solve a problem could often be traced to poor problem statement, owing to inexperience, lack of knowledge or reliance on the medical model.

Aspinall (1976), on the other hand, showed that experienced nurses (with more than ten years' clinical experience) also failed to recognise problems and the relationship between problems. She suggested that it was nurses' traditional education which caused them to behave in this way. Corcoran (1986) has gone further. She tested expert and novice nurses and found that: (1) both novices and experts failed to recognise important problems; (2) experts failed to record and subsequently forgot problems, owing to limitations of their short-term memory; and (3) novices over-simplified patients' problems, owing to a lack of knowledge and experience. Following a detailed study of the theory and practice of the nursing process de la Cuesta (1983) reported that nurses found difficulty stating nursing problems and dismissed relevant problems. Although the differences between novice and expert nurses shown here are significant, the earlier warning regarding the confounding effect of the research context (p. 16) may apply to these studies; for Aspinall, Corcoran and de la Cuesta conducted their research in different settings.

Despite the importance attached to problem identification by some writers, the little amount of empirical work has shown that nurses of all levels of experience may fail to identify important problems. The reason given for this failure is mainly inexperience, although the sequence of the nursing process may also be to blame. As we have seen, problem identification is not given individual status, but is incorporated within the assessment stage of most accounts of the nursing process. This practice may influence the nurse's thinking.

2. Problem assessment

Problem assessment means collecting, estimating and judging the value
and significance of data for the patient's care (Vitale et al., 1978, p. 87;
Lauri, 1982). This assessment is a deeper, problem-specific, systematic and
formal collection of data, rather than the more generalised process
associated with problem identification (Johnson et al., 1980, pp. 56–7).

Assessment enables the nurse to understand the problem further, judge
the extent of the problem and trace the relationship between problems
(Vitale et al., 1978, pp. 38–46). It is claimed to be a crucial step in clinical
problem-solving because it is the basis for any planned nursing intervention
(Wooley et al., 1974, p. 68; Barker, 1987).

This second stage helps to break down the problem into sub-problems
and find their causes. Not surprisingly, it may lead to the discovery of fresh
problems (Priestley et al., 1979, p. 21; Barker, 1987). Assessment, like
problem identification, can involve the patient, his or her relatives, or
other health-care workers (Johnson et al., 1980, p. 47; Lauri, 1982).

Assessment depends on the nurse's skills and knowledge, particularly
the ability to communicate with the patient, and the capacity to select
relevant material. The nurse also needs to use interviewing and decision-
making skills to conduct the assessment. These skills and knowledge help
to build a profile of the patient (see Hammond, 1966; Vitale et al., 1978,
pp. 38–46; Barker, 1987). As in the case of problem identification, an
incomplete assessment may be due to lack of knowledge, poor data
collection and classification (Aspinall, 1976; Johnson et al., 1980, p. 72;
Corcoran, 1986).

Despite the primacy of problem assessment, particularly in the nursing
literature, the relationship between problem identification and problem
assessment is confused. As Table 2.1 shows, some stages models begin
with problem identification before moving on to problem assessment (e.g.
Beeler, 1987; others start with problem assessment without reference to a
problem identification stage (e.g. Hollingworth, 1985). Greaves (1987), on
the other hand, uses an intermediary 'problem definition' stage between
problem identification and problem assessment. One reason for the
differences between stages models is that some models are merely speculative with no empirical base. The situation requires clarification for nurse
education and practice.

3. Planning interventions

The planning stage of clinical problem-solving follows and is dependent on
the quality of the nursing assessment of the patient (McCarthy, 1981). The
nursing plan is a written statement of the patient's nursing problems and

the measures which will be used to effect a solution (Johnson et al., 1980, p. 78). Nursing plans need to be both tentative and flexible because of the dynamic state of the patient's health and nursing needs. They do, however, help to prioritise the patient's care (Vitale et al., 1978, pp. 8–9). The main purpose of the plan is to help the patient reach a major goal such as a return as near as possible to his or her previous health state (Kron, 1966, p. 141).

The goals are the central feature of the planning stage (Johnson et al., 1980, p. 78). Like the problem, goals should be expressed in concise, precise, measurable, patient-oriented and positive terms. Goals may need to be prioritised in line with the patient's problems (Johnson et al., 1980, pp. 75–85; Lauri, 1982). Barnett (1985, p. 25), for example, writes:

> I have found the most practical way is to write nursing goals in terms of the expected or desired change I hope to achieve with the patient. If these are written as a description of the change or outcome in terms specific to the patient, the evaluation stage of the nursing process cycle is much easier to accomplish . . . . If the patient's problem is clearly described in terms specific to the individual patient, then the goal description follows in specific terms much more easily.

There is, however, some evidence to suggest that nurses, especially less experienced nurses, have particular difficulty with articulating clear and realistic goals which may lead to a failure to solve the problem (Barnett, 1985). As we have seen in problem identification and problem assessment, and now in the planning stage, a nurse's knowledge and experience are emerging as important variables in clinical problem-solving (Vitale et al., 1978, p. 12).

The other component of planning is the selection of nursing interventions to achieve goals. Goals require action, and the nurse has to choose from a list of alternative strategies the one which has the greatest chance of attaining the goal (Bailey and Claus, 1975, pp. 25–6).

The importance of the plan to nursing practice in terms of the nurse working as an autonomous practitioner has been emphasised (Hammond, 1966; McCarthy, 1981). On the other hand, nursing plans may also include medical treatments which also contribute to goal achievement (Johnson et al., 1980, p. 78). But the need to retain medical interventions within the nursing plan may prevent nursing practice from becoming completely autonomous.

The written plan is an important record because it is the means of communicating information to other carers (Vitale et al., 1978, p. 72; de la Cuesta, 1983). Recording and storing nursing data are also important for future reference, particularly in the case of medical–legal inquiries (Barnett, 1985).

Barnett's statement on the planning stage (1985, p. 25) suggests that the patient's agreement to the plan is implicit when he or she is involved in drawing it up. The patient's relatives and other health professionals may also be involved in the planning process and help the nurse to solve the problems (Vitale et al., 1978, pp. 8–9; Johnson et al., 1980, pp. 78–9). The present author, however, feels that the patient's involvement in the planning stage is an ideal that may be difficult to achieve in some cases because the patient may not have the strength or knowledge to contribute. After all, the nurse who favours patient involvement is expecting the patient to have an understanding of health care that nurses have taken months or even years to develop. Nevertheless, the nurse should recognise the patient's contribution to planning and assess his or her capabilities in this respect.

Planning, as with the other stages, is felt to be an important step in the model. Yet despite a wide search of the literature, including the more recent work, very few of the articles and books consulted provided empirical evidence on nurses' planning strategies. The problem is highlighted in an article by Hardy and Engel (1987), who criticise nursing plans for hampering nurses' thinking. It is difficult to support or refute this criticism without adequate empirical evidence.

4. Implementation

Implementing the plan means that the nurse and other carers perform activities for and with the patient to accomplish the goals set by the nurse (Johnson et al., 1980, pp. 87–8). At face value, it seems that this stage is composed largely of practical nursing skills, but implementing the plan includes intellectual activities too. The nurse has to decide which part of the plan takes priority, who would be the best person to carry out nursing actions, which procedures and policies are involved, and what time can be devoted to the care in view of other patient demands (Vitale et al., 1978, pp. 83–7). Once again, nursing knowledge and experience are important when making these decisions as Johnson et al. (1980, p. 87) illustrate:

> It is no easy task to implement a plan of care for one patient and most nurses care for more than one patient. During the nursing education process the student first learns to create and implement one plan and then gradually increases the number of patients for whom she can manage care. As nursing knowledge and experience grows the nurse is able to plan and implement care for more complex problems and a larger number of problems concurrently.

The authors then list the required skills, gained through experience, to implement the nursing plan successfully.

There are conflicting views and evidence in the literature on planning and implementation. As mentioned earlier, considerable importance is attached to the planning process. However, Miller (1984), when evaluating the effect of the nursing process on the quality of patient care, observed that nurses failed to practise the nursing actions advocated by the plan. This indicates that writing a plan, in some cases, may be merely a routine procedure, and the content may be ignored.

Given that implementation was cited 44 times in the 55 stages models reviewed, its importance in the problem-solving process is paramount. It is interesting to note, however, that the amount written about this stage in both the general and nursing literature tends to be less than that written about the other stages. The present author feels that the principal reason for this may be that implementation tends to be seen as a mechanical act, particularly in nursing. Also, the physical and intellectual actions associated with implementation tend to be discussed in an anecdotal way, and largely lack supporting evidence.

5. Evaluation

Evaluation is the stage of clinical problem-solving that helps to foster the desired outcome by checking and, if necessary, adjusting the other stages (Kron, 1966, p. 60; Vitale et al., 1978, pp. 83–5). Moreover, as the patient's health-state changes, so new nursing problems appear, which call for a continual evaluation of nursing actions (Johnson et al., 1980, pp. 97–102; Lauri, 1982).

Although evaluation is the last stage of problem-solving, it is not the final one. Rather, it is the completion of a cycle of activities, the results of which have a continuing effect upon the other stages (Priestley et al., 1979, p. 118; Pont, 1986). Successful nursing actions may indicate a need for reassessment of the patient for identification of fresh problems as a result of changes in health-state (Johnson et al., 1980, pp. 97–8). Unsuccessful strategies, however, call for an evaluation of why and where things went wrong – for example, failure to reach a solution may have been caused by inappropriate goals. The process is then restarted at that point and continued until the problem is solved (Johnson et al., 1980, pp. 97–102; Pont, 1986). Thus evaluation serves three main purposes: (1) it is a check on how far a goal has been achieved; (2) it provides a check on whether the problem has been solved; and (3) it provides feedback on the effectiveness of the nursing strategy for future reference (Ashworth and Castledine, 1981; Waters, 1986).

The skills required by the nurse during this stage are the same as those required in the assessment stage: mainly observation and judgement (Bailey and Claus, 1975, pp. 105–10; Pont, 1986). It is also important, as with the other stages of problem-solving, that the patient's view is considered (McCarthy, 1981).

Evaluation was the most frequently cited stage in both nursing and other literature covering the stages models of problem-solving (Table 2.2).

Despite the importance attached to evaluation, there is evidence to suggest that it is the least understood and possibly the least used stage in clinical problem-solving (Waters, 1986). In her study of the nursing process, de la Cuesta (1983, p. 369) found that 'Although nurses occasionally asked for feedback on the task performed, overall nursing care was not evaluated, either in written records, or during the report sessions'. In discussing some reasons for this weakness de la Cuesta states that it is difficult to hold one nurse accountable for a patient's care when several nurses are contributing to that care. Frederickson and Mayer (1977) noted that evaluation was not often used by learner nurses, and they concluded that the individuals' lack of knowledge and inexperience was the main reason for an incomplete evaluation. Vitale et al. (1978, p. 85) noted another difficulty with evaluation: some nurses use the term evaluation and assessment interchangeably.

Criticisms of the stages model theory in nursing

Although much of the literature supports the stages model theory of problem-solving in nursing, there are a number of notable criticisms. Many of these centre on the nursing process, and there is an implicit demand for further articulation and/or research, as Chenitz and Swanson (1984, pp. 205–6) explain:

> Nursing process consists of those problem-solving actions and interactions between nurse and client that are directed toward a specific end. These goal-directed behaviours are the ways in which nurses carry out the basic nursing process . . . However, the numerous applications of the basic nursing process used by nurses in daily practice cannot capture the level of sophistication and the complexity that explains and predicts what nurses do and why, until systematic articulation of the nursing process is done . . . It is essential that we attend to this task, since the basic nursing process has already been defined and analysed, yet the sub-processes that compose this process are lacking.

Hardy and Engel (1987, p. 38), in similar vein, present other criticisms:

> The adoption of one method of problem solving may not confer a cloak of respectability, rather it may reveal more about nursing as a static profession. In the past 20 years, the world has changed drastically, yet the nursing process has been clung to tenaciously. Is this because it works well or because too much money has been invested in it to let go and explore other methods? . . . The nursing process came into fashion when assumptions were made that nurses' problem-solving skills were inadequate.

They go on to explain that the stages model works well in a nursing education context, but in a clinical setting it reduces the patient to a number of problems. They prefer a more holistic approach to the provision of individualised care.

Another concern is that a nurse's problem-solving style may be idio-syncratic; that is, he or she may use a different problem-solving strategy for similar problems in different situations and, therefore, a general model like the stages model is not appropriate for the many varied situations that a nurse is likely to encounter (Bailey and Claus, 1975, Chapter 1). Both Hardy and Engel (1987) and Tanner et al. (1987), for example, point out that nurses' problem-solving strategies are not linear, but can change from problem to problem, depending on the situation. In short, it would seem that the stages model theory of problem-solving in nursing is a well-supported but under-researched aspect of nursing (Westfall et al., 1986).

So far, attention has been given to problem-solving in nursing. It is now appropriate to extend the review of the literature to look at problem-solving in other disciplines for comparative purposes. Some writers discuss theories of problem-solving in one discipline in relation to another. Yeaw (1979), for example, attempts to bridge the gap between clinical nursing and nurse education by using a stages model theory of problem-solving as a bond. Burton (1979, pp. 7–14) and Hill (1979, pp. 15–139) consider problem-solving in many educational settings and disciplines related to education; while McCarthy (1981) compares and contrasts clinical problem-solving in nursing and medicine. It is suggested that practitioners, teachers and researchers in one speciality can learn from problem-solving research undertaken elsewhere.

The next chapter examines the problem-solving process in medicine, management and education. The disciplines chosen are ones in which nurses operate for at least part of their professional role. Medicine was selected because of the strong clinical relationship between medical and nursing practice; management because it is both taught and practised by nurses; and education because of its importance to the development of nurses and nursing.

4

Problem-solving in Related Disciplines

An examination of the problem-solving literature on the related disciplines to nursing, namely medicine, management and education, reveals many similarities and some differences.

Problem-solving in medicine

Medical problem-solving is a process of making an 'accurate diagnosis' and a 'management plan' for the individual patient with the intention of improving health (Vu, 1979, p. 282; Berner, 1984, p. 626). As in nursing, problem-solving in medicine is discussed in the literature in terms of the two main theories: information-processing system and the stages model theories (Elstein et al., 1978, Chapter 2; McGuire, 1985), with the emphasis on the former. Other, less well-documented interpretations include the clinical judgement approach and the decision-analysis/ probability model (McGuire, 1985).

Despite the emphasis in the medical literature on the information-process system theory, it is agreed that no one theory is appropriate to all medical problems (see Elstein et al., 1978, Chapter 2; Harasym et al., 1979, p. 67; Neufeld et al., 1981; McGuire, 1985; Holzemer, 1986).

It appears that much more of the medical problem-solving literature is empirically-based than is the case in nursing, but McGuire (1985) believes that the research is limited because of poor research design in some cases. Indeed, Elstein et al. (1978, pp. 275–6) criticise some of this work by pointing out sampling, validity and reliability weaknesses. The process of problem-solving in medicine will now be examined in terms of information-processing and stages models.

Information-processing system theory in medical problem-solving

Newell and Simon's original work (1972) on human problem-solving is used in medicine to explain the actions physicians employ when interacting with a patient. Elstein et al. (1978, Chapter 11), in an extensive analysis of medical problem-solving, claim to have used an eclectic approach, but their work is based mainly on the information-processing system theory. In their analysis, full use is made of all three aspects of the theory, namely the task environment (pp. 175–84), the problem space (pp. 175–6) and the problem-solving strategies (pp. 180–98). The problem space, in a medical context, is explained in much the same way as in the original work of Newell and Simon (1972, pp. 59–80). It is the physician's representation of the problem constructed from perceptions of the patient's illness, and knowledge of and experience with similar situations which are adapted to the present task (McGuire, 1985). The physician's problem space has an overwhelming influence on the problem-solving strategy adopted; that is, it determines how the problem will be tackled (Elstein et al., 1978, pp. 150–1).

More specifically, the problem space is made up of one or more problem formulations (Elstein et al., 1978, p. 176) or 'diagnostic impressions' (McGuire, 1985), which are more commonly referred to as diagnostic hypotheses (Elstein et al., 1978, p. 169). The hypothesis may be the diagnosis of a disease, a syndrome, a pathological process or a psychological concept (Feightner et al., 1977). Neufeld et al. (1981) explain that the construction of diagnostic hypotheses is a key activity and a major aid to medical problem-solving. Selecting and analysing hypotheses helps the physician to simplify the task of treating a patient, because it limits the size of the problem space and the subsequent search for a solution (Elstein et al., 1978, pp. 277–8).

Following the initial encounter with the patient, the physician begins to generate several diagnostic hypotheses (Neufeld et al., 1981). It is suggested that this is an exercise in pattern-matching, where the physician compares his or her immediate observations with knowledge of similar experiences, selecting the hypotheses which best fit the assessment of the patient (Feightner et al., 1977; McGuire, 1985).

Errors in diagnosis may be avoided by arranging the hypotheses in a hierarchical fashion and then systematically eliminating those lacking supporting evidence. It is interesting that apparently more time is spent confirming hypotheses than refuting them (Feightner et al., 1977). Gathering data to confirm or refute each hypothesis may arise from a physical examination, or laboratory and radiological tests (Neufeld et al., 1981).

The search for supporting evidence moves from a known point to a specified goal. One of the more common search strategies is means–ends analysis, where the physician concentrates on a cluster of findings and then reduces the distance from the actual state to the desired state. In this way, the physician uses hypotheses to aid the search for confirmatory evidence (Elstein et al., 1978, p. 114). Another strategy, 'generate and test', includes the listing of hypotheses in a hierarchical fashion, deciding on the interrelatedness of clues before selecting the final diagnosis (Feightner et al., 1977).

An interesting point is that despite the inclusion of the terms 'treatment' and 'management plan' in some definitions of medical problem-solving (Feightner et al., 1977, p. 67; Elstein et al., 1978, p. 273; Berner, 1984, p. 626), there is very little mention in the literature of patient management within the medical problem-solving process. That is, the implementation and evaluation of treatment to overcome the medical problem is rarely discussed. It would appear, therefore, that the major activity is to achieve a correct diagnosis. McGuire (1985, p. 590), writing about 'labelling', noted that:

> careful analysis of the tasks . . . physicians are typically directed to perform suggests they are usually asked to label something and not solve a problem. Though most investigators would probably agree that labelling and problem solving are not identical cognitive processes, they generally report their studies in a manner which strongly implies that the so-called problem has been solved once the correct label (that is, diagnosis) has been attached to it.

Elstein et al. (1978, p. 273), while not dismissing the treatment process, also emphasise the importance of diagnostic reasoning in their investigation into medical problem-solving:

> The focus of this study is largely on the processes of diagnostic reasoning, although questions of treatment selection and management are also addressed. . . . However, we believe that rationality is desirable and necessary in medicine, although it is by no means sufficient, and that it is therefore worthwhile to understand diagnostic reasoning.

However, once the diagnosis has been made, it is followed by the application of a standard solution in the form of medical or surgical treatment (Vu, 1979; Berner, 1984), but it would seem that treatment, obviously a major activity in medicine, is not considered to be a problem-solving activity. One possible reason for the concentration on diagnostic problem-solving is that the medical model, as we saw earlier (p. ix), assumes a non-individualised approach to patient care in the sense that a standard treatment is applied to an illness which has been accurately diagnosed.

Stages model theory in medical problem-solving

Although, as mentioned earlier, there is an obvious emphasis on the information-processing system theory in the literature on medical problem-solving, curiously, when it comes to summarising or generalising research findings, writers tend to use a stages model (McGuire, 1985). This can be seen in Elstein et al. (1978, p. 277). They begin by indicating the complexity of medical problem-solving, but end with a four-stage model of problem-solving to help the reader's understanding:

> Although differences in the content of the memory store apparently distinguish stronger from weaker problem-solving performance, this does not imply that medical problem solving is dependent solely upon mastery of passively recalled content. Knowledge must be retrieved and organised. Medical problems typically require that additional data be gathered and evaluated. Ill-defined problems must be progressively better defined so that rational action can be taken. Alternative interpretations of probabilistic data must be generated and compared. These activities are summarized in a four-stage general model of medical inquiry that calls attention to cue acquisition, hypothesis generation, cue interpretation, and hypothesis evaluation.

Stages models feature particularly in the literature on medical education (Joorabchi, 1981; Cox and Ewan, 1982, pp. 94–101; McGuire, 1985). One reason for this appears to be a need to represent a difficult topic in a simple way, helping the writer to explain an activity which is not easily described, and the reader to understand the complex issues of problem-solving (Forehand, 1966, p. 362; Elstein et al., 1978, Chapter 11). Medical students may need the step-by-step approach of a stages model to help their understanding of the diagnostic problem-solving process. However, as we have seen (pp. 12), Forehand (1966, p. 362) argues strongly that problem-solving is not a step-wise process. It would seem, therefore, that some medical and nursing writers disregard the principles of the information-processing system theory.

As a result of the tendency to use the stages model to summarise the medical problem-solving process, there is very little detailed discussion of each element of this model. It certainly does not approach the level of discussion found in the nursing literature, or indeed the education and management literature. The following stages model, consisting of the four elements described by Vu (1979, p. 282), is typical of others to be found in the medical literature:

1. data collection;
2. interpretation of data;
3. hypothesis generation;
4. evaluation.

We can see that this model bears only a slight resemblance to the stages models described in the nursing literature; this is because the main goal in medical problem-solving is to arrive at an accurate diagnosis, and planning and implementation are omitted. Nurses and doctors both attempt to identify the problem, but nurses go on to devise a plan, implement it and evaluate the intervention in an effort to resolve the problem. Diagnostic hypotheses do not appear to feature in the UK nursing literature on problem-solving, but seem to be discussed much more in the literature from North America (Holzemer, 1986; Tanner et al., 1987).

From the evidence reviewed so far, writers tend to favour the information-processing system theory as an interpretation of medical problem-solving. It is believed to be a process consisting of the formulation and confirmation of diagnostic hypotheses based on an assessment of the patient and an analysis of other related data. The key processes appear to be the formation of diagnostic hypotheses (the problem space) and the collection of data to confirm hypotheses (the problem-solving strategy). It is a labelling process, rather than a treatment process. Finally, medical problem-solving is thought to be case-specific rather than something that can be generalised to all medical problems.

Problem-solving in management

A managerial problem is a gap between an actual state and a desired state. Problem-solving in management, therefore, is a process of identifying and justifying solutions in a systematic question-posing way to close the gap and solve the problem (see Margerison, 1974, pp. 19–22; Kaufman, 1982, p. 12; Greenwood et al., 1983, p. 12). An effective solution to a managerial problem is cost-effective, reliable, efficient, adaptable and acceptable to those who have to implement it (Margerison, 1974, p. 31).

Managerial problem-solving covers a large area, including financial, personal, economic and health-care problems (Greenwood et al., 1983, pp. 27–88). For the purposes of this book, the literature review and subsequent discussion of managerial problem-solving has been limited to interpersonal problem-solving, in line with nursing, medicine and education.

Management problems tend to be open-ended and ill-defined. This is because these problems are often conflict-oriented and include goals which are complex, ill-structured and have a shifting quality owing to the number of variables involved (Shone, 1974, p. 33; Greenwood et al., 1983, p. 12; Simon et al., 1987). As we have seen, the type of problem is an important determinant of the way an individual, in this case a manager, solves a problem (Simon et al., 1987).

Managerial problem-solving can be either multidisciplinary, that is a committee-based activity, or handled by an individual (Greenwood et al., 1983, pp. 14–24; Marriner-Tomey, 1988, p. 87). In the case of the problem-solving strategies of individual managers, several approaches are described in the literature. For example, Gillis (1983, pp. 23–5) categorises strategies as 'traditional', 'rational', 'experimental' and 'creative', while Margerison (1974, p. 13) uses a broader classification of 'problem-centred' and 'solution-centred' problem-solving. As in other disciplines, the more detailed descriptions include the information-processing system theory (Simon et al., 1987) and the stages model theory (Shone, 1974, pp. 21–32; Greenwood et al., 1983, pp. 25–7; Marriner-Tomey, 1988, pp. 220–4).

Information-processing system theory in managerial problem-solving

Generally speaking, the application and discussion of the information-processing system theory in the management literature has, as its basis, the original work of Newell and Simon (1972) and the more recent work of Simon et al. (1987).

The manager represents the problem as a problem space, which is made up of goals and a network of information (Simon et al., 1987). He or she then reduces the problem space using heuristics or rules of thumb to guide the search for a solution. Two heuristics in particular are described. The first, sometimes referred to as 'hill climbing', is one whereby the manager uses one goal to determine where it would be most profitable to look next in the search for a solution (Simon et al., 1987), in the way a climber would progress up a rock face. The second heuristic, sometimes known as means–ends analysis is the one more commonly used. Here, the solver compares the present situation with a goal, detects a difference between them, and then calls on existing knowledge to reduce the distance between the actual state and the desired state. As Simon et al. (1987, p. 21) explain:

> Thus, if the difference is a 50 mile distance from the goal, the problem solver will retrieve from memory knowledge about autos, carts, bicycles, and other means of transport; walking and flying will probably be discarded as inappropriate for that distance.

Boreham (1986) sees things differently. He suggests that the problem-solving strategy is mainly one of asking questions to search for data that will support or refute one or more hypotheses set by the manager early in the problem encounter. Boreham goes on to explain that the solution is recognised by a mixture of pattern recognition and intuition.

Despite the work of Boreham (1986) and Simon et al. (1987), research into the information-processing system approach to managerial problem-solving is felt to be inadequate (Simon et al., 1987). The initial actions in this type of problem-solving, in particular how the manager frames the problem, are poorly understood, as Simon et al. (1987, p. 24) point out:

> The very first steps in the problem-solving process are the least understood. What brings (and should bring) problems to the head of the agenda? And when a problem is identified, how can it be represented in a way that facilitates its solution?

It is interesting to note that this fairly recent quotation comes from an acknowledged expert on information-processing systems and problem-solving, who suggests there is a lack of understanding in this area, and thus poor understanding of the problem space. A reduced understanding of how the problem space is constructed affects what is known about problem-solving strategies.

Stages model theory in managerial problem-solving

This theory is a popular approach to explaining, teaching and learning problem-solving within the discipline of management (Kaufman, 1982, p. 154). Shone (1974, p. 21) is particularly supportive of this model:

> Problem solving is difficult and does require hard thinking . . . This is done by splitting a whole activity or problem into a series of consecutive steps. There are several advantages in doing this. First it gets over the impossibility of thinking of many things simultaneously . . . Secondly it avoids the situation in which thinking gravitates around but never strikes into a problem.

Kaufman (1982, p. 154) suggests that stages models are excellent bridge-builders between the problem and its solution. Others suggest that the logical, step-wise and cyclical method of the stages model lessens the chance of a manager making errors and improves cost-effectiveness (Shone, 1974, pp. 21–32; Greenwood et al., 1983, pp. 12–26). Other writers (e.g. Crout, 1987) favour this method because it has a universal quality, in that it can be applied to many managerial problems.

As in the case of the stages models discussed so far, the names of elements in the several models in the management literature vary. The stages model below, described by Greenwood et al. (1983, pp. 25–6), is similar to the one the researcher derived from the general literature (Table 2.4) and is also representative of others in the management literature:

1. identifying the type of problem faced;
2. analysing the problem;
3. decision-making;
4. decision-taking – implementation;
5. outcome evaluation.

Managerial problems are identified from the needs of an organisation, and it is claimed that successful management depends on accurate problem identification (Kaufman, 1982, p. 96; Greenwood et al., 1983, pp. 14–15; Marriner-Tomey, 1988, pp. 4–5).

Problem analysis helps the manager to identify the cause of the problem and the events leading up to it. Managerial problem-solving is strengthened by the addition and consideration of quantitative data (Shone, 1974, pp.

24–34; Greenwood et al., 1983, p. 19). Problem analysis calls for many skills, including judgement, decision-making, careful observation and skilful questioning (Kaufman, 1982, p. 97; Greenwood et al., 1983, pp. 16–17).

The middle-order stages (decision-making and taking) include the setting of clear and measurable objectives and the development of a strategy to meet the objectives. Objective-setting is felt to be crucial, particularly in providing a yardstick for the evaluation stage (Greenwood et al., 1983, pp. 17–21; HCEA, 1987, p. 70; Marriner-Tomey, 1988, pp. 4–7).

The last stage in managerial problem-solving is an analysis of how effective the chosen course of action has been in meeting the manager's objective (HCEA, 1987, p. 70). It is suggested that there are two types of evaluation: the first is the identification of factors which led to the successful outcome for the purpose of self-learning; the second helps determine why the outcome has not been successful so that corrective action can be taken (Greenwood et al., 1983, p. 22). Evaluation seems to have an extended role in managerial problem-solving. The manager not only judges the success or failure of the strategy, but also determines what stage was particularly successful or unsuccessful for future reference (Margerison, 1974, pp. 30–47; HCEA, 1987, p. 71). Evaluation may also be used to highlight the cost-benefit element of managerial problem-solving, that is, the cost of a strategy compared with the usefulness of the outcome (Marriner-Tomey, 1988, p. 7). As a result, quantitative measures may need to be taken in the evaluation stage (Greenwood et al., 1983, pp. 22–4).

However quick the process, a step-wise model of problem-solving can help the manager make fewer mistakes (Greenwood et al., 1983, p. 24). But with reference to the problem-solving stages, Shone (1974, pp. 21–31) makes an unusual suggestion that has not been encountered elsewhere in the literature. He suggests that certain steps in the problem-solving process may be removed to improve problem-solving efficiency.

Other approaches to managerial problem-solving

Apart from the information-processing system and stages model theories of problem-solving, there are other approaches of some importance. For example, Margerison (1974, pp. 14–33) argues that managerial problem-solving is either problem-centred or solution-centred. The emphasis in problem-centred behaviour is on the search for relevant information which is felt to be an important managerial skill. The emphasis in solution-centred behaviour is on the development and advancement of ideas which aim to solve the problem. This approach is only appropriate when the manager has identified the problem and has a solution which has merit and acceptability for all concerned.

He goes on to describe two problem-centred and three solution-centred approaches.

Problem-centred approaches:
1. consultative-oriented, where the manager generates and shares knowledge about the problem by discussing the problem with subordinates;
2. reflective-oriented, in which the manager uses a non-directive, listening and advising approach. Here, an attempt is made to persuade subordinates to 'own' the problem.

Solution-centred approaches:
1. directive-oriented, where the manager tells others what is to be done. He or she takes a direct line by issuing an order. Although this approach has a place in management, it tends to be played down by managers;
2. prescriptive-oriented, where the manager advises what should be done. This is a common approach, but its success depends on the subordinate's trust in the manager's judgement;
3. negotiative-oriented, where the manager seeks compliance from subordinates in return for a reward. This form of bargaining is a well-recognised style of management in industry.

It is suggested that the manager may use one or more of these approaches when solving a problem. Margerison (1974) explains that these strategies have particular relevance to management–worker relations, and cites several vignettes in which they have worked. It is clear, however, that they are broad-brush methods, which do not articulate the finer points of the problem-solving process, seen, for example, in Greenwood et al.'s (1983) model. Margerison's model would, however, serve as a useful framework for managers dealing with problems arising between the manager and employees.

To summarise, the process of problem-solving in management is almost a reversal of that found in the medical literature, but very similar to that found in nursing. That is, the stages model theory seems to dominate the literature. One reason for this is that the stages model is flexible and can be applied to the diverse range of problems likely to be encountered by a manager. The stages model also fits well in the cost–benefit emphasis in some types of management. One main reason why the information-processing system theory does not feature strongly in this literature is the predominance of ill-defined problems in management. A second reason, as Simon et al. (1987) point out, is the lack of research in this area.

Problem-solving in education

The literature on problem-solving in education shares common features with health-care and management problem-solving literature. First, it has a strong interpersonal element, and second, it reflects the same division between the information-processing system and the stages model theories (see Schmuck et al., 1966; Hill, 1979; Tuma and Reif, 1980). In addition, there is Schön's unique and innovative work in his *Educating the Reflective Practitioner* (1987).

The process of problem-solving in education is seen as (1) facilitating teaching and learning (Schmuck et al., 1966, p. 1), (2) acquiring problem-solving skills (Hill, 1979, pp. 85–100) and (3) understanding the cognitive processes involved (Stewart, 1985; Garrett, 1986). But the process of problem-solving in education is still unclear (Hill, 1979, pp. 15–16). As Garrett (1986, p. 90) explains:

> the whole field of endeavour in problem solving is particularly vast and largely disorganised . . . we are as removed from an understanding of the process of problem solving and its relationship to solver and task variables as we have ever been.

This may, in part, be the result of the individual differences learners show in problem-solving and the influence of the educational setting upon the problem (Garrett, 1986). Those attempts which have been made to explain the process of problem-solving in education are now discussed.

Information-processing system theory in educational problem-solving

The information-processing system theory is playing an increasing role in the understanding of problem-solving in the classroom (Tuma and Reif, 1980; Whitman, 1983; Stewart, 1985). Once again, much of the discussion centres on the formulation of the problem space and the heuristics used to reach a solution (Tuma and Reif, 1980, pp. 81–95). More specifically, Stewart (1985) and Garrett (1986) believe that a major variable in the structure of the problem space and problem-solving strategies is the solver's knowledge and experience. Stewart (1985) divides knowledge into (1) conceptual knowledge important to the way the problem is perceived, and (2) strategic knowledge, which governs the heuristics the solver will employ in the problem space. In an educational setting, it is both the conceptual knowledge of the discipline and the procedural knowledge related to the problem that will determine the problem space, the heuristics used, and the speed and accuracy of problem-solving.

Larkin (1980, pp. 117–20) and Stewart (1985), in their studies of science education, go on to say that novices have different problem-solving strategies from experts. Novices' problem-solving is characterised by the manipulation of smaller chunks of information, by the setting of goals and sub-goals, and by frequent checks on progress through feedback. Experts, on the other hand, use a more global approach because of their ability to organise concepts and in particular their use of well-known search strategies such as means–end analysis. Also, in some situations, experts tend to reorganise the problem before employing heuristics. It is apparent that the study of expert and novice problem-solving is not as detailed in other disciplines as it is in education.

Stages model theory in educational problem-solving

Schmuck et al. (1966) have examined problem-solving in the classroom in detail. Their interpretation is based solely on the stages model theory and provides convincing arguments, supplemented with several classroom vignettes, for its use in education.

Schmuck et al. begin by explaining that teachers are constantly faced with classroom problems, which can be dealt with in many ways. Teachers may use one of the following 'problem-solving styles' (Schmuck et al., 1966, p. 6):

1. problem denial, where the teacher lacks insight into the problem, or energy to tackle it;
2. authoritarian problem-solving, where solutions are enforced without logical rationale;
3. least-effort problem-solving, where little work is put into dealing with a problem;
4. personal satisfaction problem-solving, where only information supporting the desired outcome is gathered;
5. pure-empiricist style, where data are used to solve the problem;
6. intuitive problem-solving, where priority is given to thought processes and reasoning;
7. empirical-rational problem-solving, where empirical data and theoretical approaches are used.

The authors feel that the first six problem-solving styles are deficient and that even the most sophisticated of them fails to make use of the instruments and data available to the teacher. They go on to recommend a stages model of problem-solving, consisting of the following steps to help improve the teacher's problem-solving skills (ibid., pp. 8–11):

1. identifying classroom problems;
2. diagnosing classroom problems;
3. developing a plan;
4. adaptation and action;
5. feedback and evaluation.

These stages are very similar to the stages model derived from the general literature. This model is an empirical-rational one because it encourages the teacher to collect relevant information by observation and by the use of diagnostic instruments, and then plan carefully and reflect upon the strategy before implementation.

The stepwise, cyclic and flexible nature of this model is emphasised. Another feature is the way it helps the teacher to clarify and simplify educational problem-solving by breaking down complex situations into more manageable parts (ibid., pp. 6–14).

Schmuck et al. (1966) describe a two-stage assessment. The first is used to identify the problem and it is felt that problem identification has a better chance of success if the teacher carefully observes and documents the observations.

Following problem identification, the teacher may then formulate hypotheses.

The second assessment is a deeper one to verify, refute or refine hypotheses. The teacher may wish to employ diagnostic instruments, or other empirical methods to assist the assessment stages. The importance here of using quantitative data, such as test data, is stressed by the authors. The collection of quantitative data was also recommended in some models in the management literature (see Margerison, 1974, pp. 24–5; Greenwood et al., 1983, p. 19).

The middle-order stages are the planning and implementation of solutions. The teacher has to decide whether an individual or group approach is required to achieve a solution. Whichever method is chosen, it is recommended that the teacher reviews the strategy before implementation. He or she may need to involve colleagues in this review process for objectivity (Schmuck et al., 1966, p. 10)

Evaluation, according to the authors, is a crucial stage in educational problem-solving and may involve learners in giving feedback to the teacher (in the case of classroom-based problems). The need to distinguish between short- and long-term evaluation is also felt to be important. Once again, it is suggested that the teacher uses quantitative data when evaluating progress and confirming the solution. Alternatively, an objective evaluation made independently by an educationalist not associated with the problem is recommended. This process helps the teacher to discover the reasons for success or failure of the problem-solving strategy. It may also result in the identification of new problems (Schmuck et al., 1966, pp. 10–11).

The stages model theory in education has proved valuable to many educationalists in that it has helped to clarify the process and made problem-solving more manageable (Hill, 1979, pp. 15–16). However, as we have seen in other disciplines, it has attracted criticism. Hill (1979, pp. 15–16), Stewart (1985) and Garrett (1986), for example, question whether the stages are identifiable activities, whether stages are testable and whether the stages model theory is generalisable to all educational problems. The information-processing system theorists have also criticised the stages model theory in this way.

The reflective practitioner

Schön (1987), in his *Educating the Reflective Practitioner*, describes an unusual model of education in which problem-solving is a key process. Schön's explanation of problem-solving is closely intertwined with his educational arguments and cannot easily be separated out. There appear to be two major differences between Schön's explanation of problem-solving and the other approaches described in this review. First, Schön's explanation is a product of the educational method suggested by him; that is, the learner's method of solving problems depends on the interaction between teacher and learner, as well as on the knowledge and experience brought to the problem situation. A second difference is the emphasis the author places upon problem-solving in a practice context, what he calls reflection-in-action – hence the title of the book. These issues will now be examined in more detail.

Schön's analysis is based largely on several case studies written to emphasise the key features of his model. In short, Schön describes problem-solving through the actions of professional practitioners who are 'thinking what they are doing while they are doing it' (1987, p. xi). As Schön explains:

> I argued for a new epistemology of practice, one that would stand the question of professional knowledge on its head by taking as its point of departure the competence and artistry already embedded in skilful practice – especially, the reflection in action . . . that practitioners sometimes bring to situations of uncertainty, uniqueness, and conflict. (Schön, 1987, p. xi)

Several important issues underpin Schön's model (pp. 3–21). He believes that when faced with a well-structured problem, the practitioner will solve the problem from experience by applying knowledge and skills gained through practice. He claims, however, that many problems in the real world are not well structured, and that it is inappropriate to use a scientific, systematic approach, typified by the stages model theory to explain the process of solving this type of problem. Instead, in the case of an ill-structured problem (an indeterminate situation), a practitioner will improvise by inventing and testing various strategies.

More specifically, Schön suggests that the practitioner selects and organises material from the problem situation, which gives direction for action. This so-called 'problem framing' is important to the problem-solving process. Practitioners frame problems in different ways because of their different knowledge and experience. For example, a dietician may concentrate on providing an optimal diet for malnourished children in developing countries, whereas a farmer may think of the problem in terms of food production, while a demographer would view it as population growth outstripping food supply. It is for these reasons that the author suggests that practitioners frame problems and shape situations to match professional understanding and methods. Problem framing is a key process, but resolution also depends on the practitioner's ability to find a solution when faced with conflicting information and inconsistencies. Once again, knowledge and experience are important to this part of the problem-solving process.

Schön describes the way a practitioner uses his or her knowledge and experience to arrive at a solution through 'reflection-in-action' (1987, pp. 63–9). This is an experimental process in which the practitioner tests and modifies his or her understanding of the problem. Schön sees finding a solution via experimentation as an important problem-solving strategy, and he describes three complementary forms of experimenting. The first is an exploration of the problem environment 'to get a feel for things' (1987, p. 70). The second is a more purposeful form of experimenting, and is intended to produce change through a process of 'move-testing' (an intended action with an end in mind) (ibid., p. 71). The third is called 'hypotheses testing' (ibid.), in which progress towards a solution is made as hypotheses are rejected and others confirmed. Schön's hypothesis-testing strategy also appears in the medical and nursing literature and plays a similar role.

To summarise, the reflective practitioner solves well-defined problems using techniques derived from experiences with similar problems. Ill-defined problems, on the other hand, are more common and are solved by a combination of processes, which include problem framing and experimentation through exploratory, move-testing and hypothesis-testing strategies.

Despite Schön's claim that his approach is different from others, there appear to be similarities between his description of problem-solving and the information-processing system theory. That is, problem framing can be equated with the notion of the problem space, and the reflection-in-action part of the problem-solving strategy is similar to some strategies described in the information-processing system theory.

The literature on educational problem-solving, taken as a whole, has several strong themes. One is the importance of problem-solving to the curriculum in that the teacher has to understand the process to facilitate teaching and learning. Another theme is the types of theory used to explain problem-solving. The literature is primarily a discussion of information-processing system and stages model theory, although Schön's work on the reflective practitioner is likely to influence future thinking. With the exception of Schön's independent stance, there is not so much a debate between educationalists as there is between the cognitive scientists regarding the appropriateness of a stages model and information-processing system. Rather, there appears to be a distinct division, which is recognised by educational researchers in that the stages model theory is often applied to the practical problems of teaching and learning, whereas the information-processing system theory is used to explain the cognitive aspects of problem-solving in education.

There are still some gaps in the knowledge of problem-solving in education (as there are in other areas), and educational researchers admit that our understanding of problem-solving is still poor. Further research is required to clarify the major issue of how ill-defined problems are solved, for example.

Issues from the review of the literature

Problem-solving in nursing appears to be considered almost exclusively as a stages model theory, whereas researchers in other disciplines sometimes attach more importance to information-processing systems, and to a lesser extent to other approaches as well. Some researchers in all areas, however, feel that the information-processing system theory may be inappropriate for real-life problems, in that it is difficult to demonstrate information-processing in the context of ill-defined problems. On the other hand, there is agreement that it provides an appropriate explanation for strategies used to solve puzzle-like problems in well-controlled conditions. Since these conditions are rarely found in nursing, this may be one reason why most nurse-researchers have not considered this theory seriously.

Perhaps the main concern is that much of the literature on nursing problem-solving is *not* based on sound empirical evidence gained from large samples; rather, it is commonly derived from personal experience, anecdotal evidence and speculation. (An example of authors who write in a speculative way is Johnson et al., 1980.) Assumptions, therefore, remain untested, some theories are relatively unsupported by empirical evidence and important questions are left unanswered. These are some of the concerns:

1. First, and perhaps most important, to what extent is the stages model a valid representation of clinical problem-solving?
2. On accepting the stages model (an assumption commonly made in the nursing literature):
   (a) Do nurses use all five elements of a typical stages model as has been questioned in the general problem-solving literature by Forehand (1966, p. 361) and Hill (1979, p. 16)?
   (b) Do nurses follow these elements in a linear fashion as some writers, including Bailey and Claus (1975, p. 10) have stated?
   (c) Are there detectable differences in the perceptions of problem-solving between experienced, newly qualified and learner nurses as McCarthy (1981), for example, would have us believe?
3. Finally, to what extent does nursing problem-solving theory compare with problem-solving theory in professions closely related to the nursing role?

Serious gaps remain in our knowledge and understanding of this field, thereby creating difficulties for nurse educators and practitioners. The strategy in this research for gaining empirical evidence to develop a theory of problem-solving in nursing is set out in the next chapter.

5

Research Design

Following a review of the literature there appeared to be a need to investigate theories of problem-solving in nursing further. The aim of this book is to contribute to this theory by systematic empirical study. The principal objectives were to:

1. investigate in depth the perceptions and understanding of nursing problem-solving demonstrated by experienced, newly qualified, and learner nurses;
2. develop a cognate theory of problem-solving in nursing;
3. compare the emergent theory with other general theories and accounts of problem-solving in the literature of nursing and allied professions.

The initial stage was an exploratory study of thirty local, experienced nurses' perceptions and understanding of clinical problem-solving. This stage was important because it enabled the author to check the feasibility of the study and its theoretical base.

After a review of the literature it became evident that either an information-processing system or a stages model could be used as a theoretical base for the study. The decision to develop and apply research instruments based on a stages model of problem-solving was mainly governed by the common practice of using a systematic approach to patient care in the United Kingdom. The decision to adopt a stages model was also based on its universal quality and ease of use in clinical problem-solving, as we have seen in Chapters 2, 3 and 4.

The subsequent stage involved interviewing a further 90 nurses with different experiences from several Health Districts to explore nurses' problem-solving in greater depth. A timetable showing the stages of the research and the main research tasks is shown in Table 5.1. The stages are discussed in more detail later in this chapter.

Table 5.1   Timetable of the main research tasks

Task	Calendar month of project
The initial stage	
Review of literature	1–8
Preparation of Vignettes 1–5	1–9
Testing vignettes	9–12
First data collection	13–21
First data analysis	21–24
The subsequent stage	
Preparation of Vignettes 6 and 7	24–27
Second data collection	27–35
Second data analysis	35–38
Writing thesis	38–

The initial stage of the study

One important aspect in the research design was deciding on an appropriate method of recording nurses' thinking processes in relation to problem-solving tasks. An inspection of the literature showed that this issue had also been carefully considered by other researchers in nursing (e.g. Jones, 1989), and by researchers in other disciplines (e.g. Elstein et al., 1978, p. 229, in medicine; Boreham, 1986, in management; and Calderhead, 1987, p. 1, in education).

Simon (1985, p. 271), Stewart (1985, p. 9) and Calderhead (1987, p. 15) explain that the methods researchers have employed to record and analyse practitioners' thinking include: (1) concurrent or retrospective verbalisation methods; (2) observation as a means of inferring practitioners' thoughts when they are at work; and (3) specially constructed interview procedures. The popularity and growth of interest in verbal protocol analysis, where subjects provide commentaries on their thinking while engaged in, for example, a problem-solving task, is evident from the expanding literature on the topic (see Chi and Glaser 1984, p. 231; Calderhead 1987, p. 5). Writers have generally commented on the strengths and weaknesses of the strategy as well as on the actual procedure.

Elstein et al. (1978, p. 287) and Calderhead (1987, p. 5) suggest that the strength of verbal protocol analysis lies in the way it enables the researcher to study a subject's cognitive processes, which are otherwise hidden from observation. It also provides the means of determining both what the problem-solver is doing and why he or she is doing it. Munro (1982, p. 53) suggests that the resultant data are a particularly rich source of the subject's sequential decision-making and data-gathering steps.

Another strength is that different stimuli can be used to elicit the subject's thoughts. For example, the stimulus could be (1) the natural interactions of the subject's work setting (Rhodes, 1984, p. 212; Calderhead, 1987, p. 5); (2) video, audio and written media (Frederickson and Mayer, 1977; Calderhead, 1987, p. 5; Jones, 1989); or (3) critical incidents (Cormack, 1984, p. 118). These methods provide the researcher with a choice, which ranges from the interfering but realistic setting (for example, the workplace) to the non-threatening but less realistic situation (for example, videos) (Munro, 1982, p. 53; Elstein et al., 1978, p. 250; Jones, 1989).

One of the weaknesses of verbal protocol analysis, as Smith (1988, p. 33) points out, is the intrusive and disruptive effect on cognitive processes of asking practitioners to think aloud. The success of the verbal protocol technique depends on the subject's ability to verbalise thoughts which are unknown to the researcher (Montague, 1982, p. 384; Kahney, 1986, p. 47). But Jones (1989) observed incidents of hesitancy, vagueness and repetition in some of her subjects who were attempting to exteriorise their thoughts during problem-solving tasks. Montague (1982, p. 384) feels that problems with self-reporting are more likely to occur when there is an element of 'the automaton' in the subject's work, where he or she may not be aware of the rationale behind the action.

Kahney (1986, p. 47) believes that some subjects report falsely in order to justify their behaviour, while others may be reticent because they feel intimidated by the researcher and/or tape recorder. In these situations, many of the subject's thoughts are unavailable for study because they remain unspoken. Subjects may also report thinking as sequential when this might not be the case, especially when retrospective analysis is taking place (Elstein et al., 1978, p. 229). Smith (1988, p. 33) also warns of the differences between data collected in natural settings (e.g. the classroom) rather than false settings (e.g. the interview room), and when the control of the process is given to the informant using, for example, conversational styles rather than structured interviews.

Several methods of collecting data were, therefore, carefully considered for this research. A decision was made to use semi-structured interviews with individual nurses, who were encouraged to comment on vignettes, rather than using methods requiring a written response from a nurse, or using observation of a practising nurse by the researcher, or using reflection on critical incidents. The use of video-taped recordings of problem-solving incidents to prompt informants seemed attractive, but was rejected because of the practical, ethical and financial implications of video recording up to seven nursing incidents. Actual observation of nurses in clinical problem-solving events was also rejected as a means of collecting data because of the difficulty of investigating nurses' thought processes at the precise time of the problem-solving incident. Questionnaires were judged unsuitable owing to their tendency to collect less in-depth data compared with interviews (Holm and Llewellyn, 1986, pp. 118–20; Polit and Hungler, 1987, p. 243).

The critical incident technique of collecting data, first described by Flanagan (1954) and used elsewhere in nursing by Cormack (1984, pp. 118–25), was also considered for this study. For example, informants could have been asked to recall clinical problem-solving incidents. This technique has the following advantages: (1) data are generated about real life events; (2) informants can reply quite easily; and (3) patients are not inconvenienced. The main disadvantages of the critical incident method are (1) the accuracy of informant's recall of events may deteriorate with the lapse of time; and (2) recall of the event is prone to selective perception (Polit and Hungler, 1987, p. 230; Marriner-Tomey, 1988, p. 119). Vignettes of clinical problem-solving were favoured over the critical incident technique because of the disadvantages or problems mentioned above. It seems, however, that the critical incident method shows promise for further in-depth empirical investigation into problem-solving.

The interview method was chosen because it enabled the researcher to collect detailed information about the informant's thoughts, perceptions, preferences, feelings and attitudes towards problem-solving, and also, to some extent, past experience of problem-solving. Interviewing allowed the researcher to clarify questions and to explore issues raised by the informant. The researcher was able to keep the discussion within the planned framework, thereby minimising the collection of irrelevant data. Another benefit was the higher response rate from interviewing compared to the use of a questionnaire (Holm and Llewellyn, 1986, pp. 118–20; Polit and Hungler, 1987, p. 243; Wilson, 1989, pp. 436–42). Audio-taping of responses allowed the researcher to concentrate on the informant's comments rather than on note taking.

It was felt that even semi-structured interviews would produce too many vague statements on problem-solving, which would be difficult to analyse. It was decided, therefore, to explore the issue of clinical problem-solving by using written vignettes as the focus of the interview. The technique of using vignettes to encourage informants to verbalise their perceptions has been used with success elsewhere (Johnson et al., 1975; Frederickson and Mayer, 1977; Elstein et al., 1978, p. 122; Munro, 1982; Baumann and Deber 1986; Putzier et al., 1986). The development and application of the vignettes used in this study are described next.

Research instruments

In the initial stage, the instruments used took the form of five written vignettes (see Appendix 1). Later, two more vignettes were added for checking purposes. Early drafts of the vignettes were tested during pilot interviews with experienced nurses and showed that, predictably, vignettes stimulated a flow of comment. The pilot study also indicated the length of time required for interviewing and whether audio-taping would be an acceptable and successful method of recording informants' perceptions for later analysis (Polit and Hungler, 1987, p. 39).

Each vignette presented a nursing problem-solving scenario based on a five-phase* model of problem-solving. It was decided to construct the scenarios with various phases deliberately omitted, and with important key words such as 'problem identification', 'assessment', 'planning', 'implementation' and 'evaluation' excluded. It was thought that this tactic would encourage nurses to reflect further on the process of problem-solving, and besides, it would be interesting to see if nurses, without prompting, detected any missing phases and/or use key words.

It was also felt that vignettes with different configurations of problem-solving phases would suit nurses' varying problem-solving styles, and that this technique would increase the chance of informants feeling comfortable with at least one vignette, thereby improving their confidence and willingness to continue.

Only one vignette (Appendix 1, no. 1) was complete, that is, it included an explanation of:

1. the way the problem was identified;
2. the way the patient was assessed;
3. the nursing plan;
4. the way the plan was implemented;
5. how the outcome was evaluated.

The other four vignettes had one or more of the phases missing, for example, Vignette 2 omitted the assessment phase. For a full list of the omissions see Table 5.2.

Each vignette was designed in such a way that it was approximately 400 words in length; contained on one page; and was capable of being read comfortably within the available time. The word-limit prevented any one vignette being visually different from the others, thereby attracting disproportionate attention. The vignettes were based on real-life incidents and were constructed from actual accounts of ward sisters' experiences documented by the author. None of the ward sisters consulted took any further part in the study.

The content of the vignettes was validated by asking more than 100 qualified nurses to judge the overall realism of the clinical problem-solving

---

* At this stage of the research 'stages model' was replaced by the term 'phase model'. It was felt that the term 'phase' better reflects the elements within the dynamic process of problem-solving in nursing, and would help to distinguish the present research model from models in other disciplines.

Table 5.2 Vignettes and their omissions

Vignette title	Phases missing
1. Miss Woods with insomnia	Nothing
2. Mr Franks, a patient who has had a partial gastrectomy	Assessment
3. Parents who complain about their child's care	Assessment and planning
4. A young man with traumatic enucleation of his left eye	Evaluation
5. Mrs Forest, a patient with ischaemic heart disease	Implementation
*6. Mr Shaw, a patient with a circulatory problem	Evaluation
*7. Mr Jones, an insulin-dependent diabetic	Planning

* Added later (see 'Subsequent Stage of the Study' for an explanation).

accounts. Each nurse provided written comments on (1) the clarity of the events; and (2) the accuracy, realism and time-scale of care and treatment. Amendments were made to each vignette, based on these comments until the final products attracted little extraneous criticism on the clinical, managerial or other procedural issues, though, naturally, criticism of omitted phases was sometimes made. This validation process sharpened up the vignettes. In total, six drafts of each vignette were constructed over a period of about nine months until a final version emerged.

The following extracts from the first draft, the third draft and the final version of Vignette 2 (Appendix 1) shows how the vignettes developed with amendments based on feedback from the nurse-validators.

First draft

A Problem-solving Scenario: Inflamed Wound
Mr Franks is 40 years old and has developed an inflamed wound three days after his partial gastrectomy for a chronic peptic ulcer. This is brought to Sister Potts' attention by Student Nurse Jones when she re-dressed the wound.

The first thing Sister Potts considers is that the patient is still ill and receiving quite intensive care and is very dependent upon the nurses for his needs. Following examination of Mr Franks' wound, Sister Potts decides to review the patient's care plan in the light of this latest development.

Following her review she tells the nurses caring for Mr Franks, Enrolled Nurse Marks and St N. Jones, of the changes to the care plan:

Care to be taken with the patient's bed bath in that he should be bathed last in case his wound is infectious. Similarly the nursing team should take care with their own hygiene. The patient's nutritional needs are being met by intravenous infusion. Once oral nutrition is recommenced the patient will be encouraged to eat a high protein diet to encourage wound healing. Furthermore, mouth care is continued to improve the patient's comfort and minimise the risk of respiratory tract infection . . .

Third draft

Vignette No. 2: Mr Franks, a Patient with an Inflamed Wound
2.1   Mr Franks is 40 years old and developed an inflamed wound three days after his partial gastrectomy for a chronic peptic ulcer. This is brought to Sister Potts' attention by Student Nurse Jones after she re-dressed Mr Franks' wound.

2.2   Sister Potts sets several goals in terms of this patient's care:

(a) to protect the other patients and staff from his possible wound infection;
(b) to improve the patient's nutritional state and encourage wound healing;
(c) to ensure that the patient remains comfortable in terms of his wound and general well-being.

2.3   Between the 3rd and 6th post-operative day Mr Franks receives the following care:

(a) one team is allocated to care for him until the suspected wound infection is confirmed or otherwise, to minimise cross-infection;
(b) the patient is soon able to tolerate oral fluids, he is then given a high protein diet to encourage wound healing;
(c) mouth care is continued to improve the patient's comfort and minimise the risk of respiratory tract infection;
(d) his vital signs are recorded 4-hourly, particular attention being paid to his body temperature;
(e) the patient's surgeon orders 'a wound swab for microscopy, culture and sensitivity' before prescribing a 7-day course of parenteral antibiotics;
(f) the wound is re-dressed daily by the same nurse and is always the last one to be re-dressed;
(g) Mr Franks and his wife are given simple explanations of the change in his care and progress;
(h) the patient's level of discomfort is assessed periodically and analgesic medication given as appropriate . . .

Final version

Vignette 2: Mr Franks, a Patient who has had a Partial Gastrectomy
2.1 Mr Franks is 40 years old and had a partial gastrectomy for a chronic peptic ulcer three days ago. Student Nurse Jones notices that the patient's wound is inflamed when changing his dressing. She covers the wound with a gauze swab and reports her worries to Sister Potts.

2.2 Sister Potts sets several goals in terms of this patient's care:

(a) to ensure that the patient remains comfortable in terms of his wound and general well-being;
(b) to improve the patient's nutritional state and encourage wound healing;
(c) to protect the other patients and staff from his possible wound infection.

2.3 Between the third and sixth post-operative day Mr Franks receives the following specific care, in addition to his general nursing care:

(a) the patient's surgeon orders 'a wound swab for microscopy, culture and sensitivity' before prescribing a 7-day course of parenteral antibiotics;
(b) the patient and his wife are given simple explanations of the change in his care and progress. They receive an initial reassurance that the inflammation will subside once the antibiotics are being received;
(c) the patient's level of discomfort is checked periodically and analgesic medication given as appropriate;
(d) one team is allocated to care for him until the result of the wound swab is known, to minimise cross-infection;
(e) the patient is soon able to tolerate oral fluids, he is then given a high-protein diet to encourage wound healing;
(f) mouth care is continued, to improve the patient's comfort and minimise the risk of respiratory tract infection;
(g) his vital signs are recorded four-hourly, particularly his temperature;
(h) the wound is re-dressed daily by the same nurse and is always the last wound to be re-dressed . . .

The validation process improved the vignettes in a number of ways. First, the differences in layout between the initial draft and final version made the latter easier to read and to reference when the informant made a specific comment. Second, the changes in language and punctuation improved the flow and clarity of the text. Third, the addition and reordering of nursing care helped to make the vignette acceptable to more informants, thereby reducing the number of critical comments from informants on relatively trivial issues. In short, as far as possible, the final version was clear, concise and clinically realistic, apart from the deliberate omissions.

None of the nurses who commented on the draft vignettes was included in the initial interview sample of 30, nor in the subsequent interview sample of 90. Elstein et al. (1978, p. 122), Munro (1982, p. 43) and Polit and Hungler (1987, p. 307) describe similar processes when developing vignettes for use in problem-solving and other research.

The sample

The selected sample needed to be as representative as possible of the nursing population under investigation (Field and Morse, 1985, pp. 37–8; Polit and Hungler, 1987, p. 222). In the initial stage of the study, it was decided to use only experienced nurses regularly involved in problem-solving, because this group was most likely to speak with authority on nursing. This sample consisted of 30 nurses who had at least two-years' post-qualification experience and comprised ward sisters, charge nurses, senior nurses and nurse teachers employed in one District Health Authority. They represented the different nursing posts, various nursing specialities and the male-to-female nurse ratio within that District.

All those asked to participate in the research appeared very interested and keen to be involved. When the informant was first approached, the author carefully explained the nature and purpose of the study. Each nurse was then given the opportunity to withdraw if he or she so wished. Informants were assured that although all the interviews would be audio-recorded, anonymity and confidentiality would be maintained. No nurse withdrew from an interview, and all interviewing was conducted by the author.

Data collection

The author maintained a consistent approach in each interview, as follows. The informant was interviewed in a quiet room where he or she first read an instruction sheet setting out the purpose and method of the interview (see Appendix 2). This was reinforced with a more detailed verbal explanation and instruction from the author (a typical introduction to an interview is given in Appendix 4).

The individual then read Vignettes 1–5, and was invited to make notes on paper provided. Following this, and after the author had answered any questions (but did not, of course, comment on the omission of any phases, or use any key words), the informant ranked Vignettes 1–5 from his or her initial impression of the problem-solving strategy. It was felt that this ranking exercise, though unimportant from a research point of view, would stimulate the informant to think about the problem-solving process displayed and should generate a framework in which to comment. It was also felt that such an easy task would enable the informant to gain confidence for the possibly more complex and demanding task ahead.

The informant was then invited to comment freely on each clinical scenario in turn and to concentrate in particular on the good and poor problem-solving actions. He or she was instructed to refer to the appropriate paragraph number when making specific comments. The informant was also given the opportunity to read each vignette again prior to the relevant discussion because of the lapse of time since it was first read.

No attempt was made to correct any errors in thinking to avoid inhibiting responses, and informants were not prompted on problem-solving issues which had not attracted their attention. The author did, however, seek clarification on some points, if this was felt appropriate (see Appendix 4 for examples of author's questions). Field and Morse (1985, pp. 66–7), in discussing interviews for research purposes, suggest that seeking clarification helps the researcher to gain the maximum value from interviews. Frederickson and Mayer (1977) used a similar method of data collection when researching nurses' problem-solving behaviour.

At the end of the session the informant was thanked for his or her time and comments. It was explained that because of the possibility of re-interview at a later date, immediate feedback could not be given, but plans for reporting the research were revealed. Finally, each person was asked not to discuss the interview with colleagues to discourage the sharing of perceptions with other likely interviewees.

Subsequent stage of the study

After a preliminary analysis of data (discussed in detail below), it became clear that planning and evaluation were not attracting as many comments as other phases (Figures 6.1–6.5). To check that this finding was not merely a consequence of the content and layout of Vignettes 3 and 4, in which planning and evaluation respectively had been omitted, two further vignettes (Vignettes 6 and 7) were written, and also omitted planning and evaluation. They were validated as described above (see p. 47) and given to informants who failed to comment on planning and evaluation in the early part of the interview.

Selection of sample

A further 60 qualified nurses (meeting the criteria of the initial sample) and 22 third-year learner and eight recently qualified nurses, the latter with experience ranging between 0 and 24 months, were added to the sample. A large sample (n = 116) was necessary to provide sufficient data for frequency counts (see Figures 6.1–6.5) and for subsequent statistical analysis (Polit and Hungler, 1987, p. 219). Extending the sample also meant that the findings would not simply reflect specific education and practice in one Health District. The larger sample also allowed a comparison to be made between learner and newly qualified nurses' perceptions of clinical problem-solving on the one hand and those of experienced nurses on the other, to see if perceptions differ with maturity. The findings may have importance when reflecting on the differences between novice and expert problem-solvers, discussed in the nursing literature (Skeet and Thompson, 1985; Corcoran, 1986; Tanner et al., 1987; Jones, 1988). The findings may also have implications for the new developments in basic and post-basic nurse education (Project 2000, UKCC, 1985; PREPP, UKCC, 1990).

For a breakdown of the employment location of the total sample see Table 5.3.

Table 5.3   The employment location of informants:
analysis by District

Health District/Board	Number
1. Central Nottinghamshire	40
2. Nottingham	17
3. North Derbyshire	10
4. Leicester	9
5. Bassetlaw	7
6. Central Manchester	4
7. Sheffield	3
8. Wakefield	3
9. North Lincolnshire	3
10. Hull	2
11. Liverpool	1
12. Durham	1
13. Scarborough	1
14. Central Birmingham	1
15. Harrogate	1
16. East Surrey	1
17. Southampton	1
18. City and Hackney	1
19. Doncaster	1
20. Dewsbury	1
21. Stockport	1
22. Gateshead	1
23. Calderdale	1
24. Burnley, Pendle and Rossendale	1
25. Barnsley	1
26. Huddersfield	1
27. Lothian	1
28. Powys	1

Informants were approached by the author after discussions with their clinical or educational manager. Most were interviewed at their place of work, but seven were interviewed during their induction programme after taking up employment in the researcher's District Health Authority following recruitment from another Health Authority.

The nurses in the subsequent stage of the study were interviewed in the same way as those in the initial sample. However, as discussed earlier, if the informant failed to discuss planning in Vignette 3 and/or evaluation in Vignette 4, then he or she was given Vignette 6 (evaluation omitted) and/ or Vignette 7 (planning omitted) to discuss.

Also, informants from the initial sample of 30, who had failed to comment on planning in Vignette 3 and evaluation in Vignette 4, were re-interviewed using the new vignettes. The author was able to conduct only 14 re-interviews from a possible 26 because some nurses were unavailable. Following the re-interviews, it was noted that of the 11 informants who failed to comment on planning in Vignette 3, eight did not discuss planning in Vignette 7. And of the 14 informants who omitted evaluation from their discussion of Vignette 4, 10 also failed to comment on evaluation in Vignette 6.

No time-limit was imposed on an interview. Each lasted approximately one hour and was audio-taped with the informant's permission, using a small, unobtrusive recorder to obtain good transcripts for protocol analysis. The informant's verbalisations provided a rich source of broad-ranging information on the process of problem-solving in nursing. However, by the time the final informants were being interviewed, no new insights were forthcoming. Data collection stopped after 116 usable interviews. Four other interviews were discarded because the informant's comments were too superficial to warrant detailed analysis.

Data analysis

Both a quantitative and qualitative approach were used to analyse the data. The results are presented in Chapters 6 and 7, respectively.

The quantitative analysis was conducted as follows. Comments connected with the recognition and non-recognition of the problem-solving phases were noted using the following categorisations applied to each transcript:

1. phase (for example, planning) present and recognised by informant;
2. phase present but no comment made by informant;
3. phase missing and omission recognised by informant;
4. phase missing but no comment made by informant.

A frequency count of recognition and non-recognition of problem identification, problem assessment, planning and evaluation was made based on this analysis, and the results are presented graphically in Figures 6.1–6.5.

Next, a frequency count of the number of occasions when each phase was discussed by informants with different levels of experience was made (see Table 6.2). Inferential statistics were then employed to investigate the differences between recognition and non-recognition of problem-solving phases. Since these data were non-parametric, the chi-square test seemed appropriate to check whether a significant difference existed between the *observed* number of respondents recognising a problem-solving phase and the number of informants *expected* to comment on the phase by chance (Wilson, 1989, p. 548). Finally, the informant's pathway through the vignette was examined to investigate the informant's thinking process (see Figure 6.6).

Qualitative analysis of interview transcripts was carried out by writing each distinct sentence or phrase onto a separate index card. The card was then coded using an interview content analysis guide (see Appendix 3). For example, comments on patient assessment were marked with an 'assessment' code 'a'. A coded, full transcript of one interview is given in Appendix 5.

The index card was also labelled with the name of the informant, his or her code number, the number of the vignette under discussion, and the statement's sequential number within the transcript. It was also possible to write comments on each card; for example, when a particular category of response was beginning to emerge which would be important for later analysis. Consequently, trends, themes and relationships in the data were summarised and described. It was decided that before a comment would be highlighted as important, at least five individual informants should make a similar comment. This method of indexing and coding transcripts made the task of cross-referencing and other data sorting more manageable.

The researcher later developed a computer program, using the principles of the card index method described above to assist the content analysis of the transcripts (Hurst et al., 1989). That is, the audio tapes were transcribed onto a computer database. One entry or record in the database became the equivalent of one index card and consisted of (1) the informant's name and interview code number; (2) the vignette number under discussion; (3) the comment and its sequential number; and (4) the content analysis code letter (as described above). The completed database comprised several thousand records, and because comments were tagged with details of the informant and vignette, etc., the program allowed the rapid printing in full of records matching selected search criteria. For example, a quest was made for informants who used 'assessment' and 'evaluation' synonymously. The computer listed seven nurses who did this, and it was found that the behaviour did not appear to be related to age, experience or any other obvious variable. The same program was also used to perform the frequency counts shown in Figures 6.1–6.5 and Tables 6.2–6.3. These analyses were completed in minutes compared with manual searches which tended to last several hours. One disadvantage, however, was that the nature of the research meant that the program had to be registered with the Data Protection Office (Data Protection Registrar, 1985).

The validity of the content analysis, used in both the manual and computer analyses was determined by asking a further 20 experienced nurses (who took no other part in the study) to analyse transcripts using the interview content analysis guide prepared by the author. This group of nurses was given a copy of:

1. the written instructions for the validation exercise;
2. the vignettes the informant was discussing (see Appendix 1);
3. a transcript of an uncoded interview with an experienced nurse (an uncoded version of Appendix 5);
4. the interview content analysis guide (see Appendix 3).

Table 6.1 shows the percentage agreement between the researcher's and independent judges' analyses. The agreement was considered to be generally satisfactory.

In summary, these analyses helped the author to describe and interpret further the informants' perceptions and understanding of clinical problem-solving. It also enabled the author to compare and contrast the relationships between the data from the study with the theoretical accounts of problem-solving in the literature for the purpose of checking and generating theory about problem-solving in nursing.

Limitations of the research design

There is no widely accepted and well-tested methodology for exploring complex issues such as the ones investigated in this research. It is wise, therefore, to point out some of the limitations of the present research design.

First, it could be argued that the phase model of clinical problem-solving was selected at the expense of the information-processing theory and the North American nursing research into diagnostic reasoning. But, as explained earlier, owing to the difficulty in applying the information-processing theory to the ill-defined problems found in nursing, it was felt that this theory would be inappropriate to use until it is better understood. In the case of diagnostic reasoning, the decision not to use this approach was based on its relative infancy at the outset of this study, and its perceived inappropriateness in the United Kingdom.

Second, although the pilot and subsequent main study showed that written vignettes of practitioners' problem-solving are a highly productive way of generating comments on problem-solving, it should be pointed out that informants were merely commenting on second-hand accounts of problem-solving. Arguably, they may have thought differently about their own problem-solving incidents. Also the content of the vignettes may have prompted informants to discuss problem-solving issues not normally considered. Furthermore, the problem-solving scenarios in the vignettes may have stifled original thought (Chi and Glaser, 1984, p. 284; Kahney, 1986, p. 47).

In order to minimise some of these problems, the researcher avoided prompting informants on problem-solving issues that had not attracted their attention. The prompts that did occur were merely intended to encourage clarification (and these were few, as can be seen in an example of a full transcript in Appendix 4).

Third, verbal protocol analysis, similar to the type used in this study, has some critics. It has been argued that asking informants to think aloud alters their thinking strategies. On the other hand, it remains a common and generally, if not universally, accepted method for analysing problem-solving processes (Elstein et al., 1978, p. 229; Hill, 1979, p. 103; Putzier et al., 1986; Westfall et al., 1986).

Fourth, Table 5.3 shows that many Districts have been undersampled and not all Districts are represented, so any generalisation of the study's findings must be tentative only. It would appear from the table that Central Nottinghamshire Health District was overrepresented, but this District was used for the initial study sample of 30 nurses as well as for the subsequent sample. An alternative strategy might have been to select a sample from one other District Health Authority equivalent to the initial first sample, rather than selecting single or small groups of practitioners from several District Health Authorities. This was not possible to arrange in the time allocated for the study, and besides, the spread of sample meant that the findings would not be unduly influenced by a District's specific nursing education and practice.

6

Nurses' Perceptions and Understanding of Clinical Problem-solving

Recognition and non-recognition of phases

The section that follows concentrates on the recognition and non-recognition of phases in clinical problem-solving. The frequency counts on which the graphs and chi-square tests are based were derived from a content analysis of each interview transcript, using the guide for analysing informants' perceptions (Appendix 3). The validity of this analysis (p. 56) was checked by asking 20 experienced nurses to carry out an analysis of the same data independently of the researcher. The percentage agreement between the researcher's analysis and the independent judges' analyses was then calculated and is given in Table 6.1. More than 50 per cent of the nurse-judges had an agreement of greater than 70 per cent. This was regarded as satisfactory.

1. Problem identification

As we saw in Table 2.2, problem identification was cited 34 times out of the 55 stages models reviewed. It seems, therefore, that problem identification is regarded as an important problem-solving activity. But is it important in nursing problem-solving?

All seven vignettes included a section on how the nurse became aware of the problem. The majority of the informants (51 per cent) mentioned actions concerning problem identification, which supports the notion that problem identification has some significance in problem-solving in nursing (Figure 6.1). A closer inspection of informants' recognition of problem identification in each vignette shows obvious differences. In only two of the seven cases was the difference between recognition and non-

Table 6.1 Percentage agreement between the researcher and independent judges' coding of one interview transcript

Independent judge	Percentage agreement
1.	91
2.	86
3.	84
4.	80
5.	78
6.	75
7.	75
8.	75
9.	73
10.	71
11.	71
12.	68
13.	67
14.	61
15.	60
16.	51
17.	51
18.	50
19.	44
20.	42

recognition of this phase statistically significant, and here there was a reversed order. In Vignette 4, the majority recognised the phase, and the difference between those who commented and those who failed to comment was statistically significant. In Vignette 5, on the other hand, the majority failed to recognise the phase, the difference again being statistically significant.

2.   Problem assessment

As we have seen, assessment is the second step in the phase of model of problem-solving derived from the literature. It is the collection of data and an analysis of the problem and sub-problems previously identified.

Figure 6.2 shows that assessment attracted comment from a high proportion of informants (71 per cent). More specifically, the highest proportion of informants who recognised assessment in any vignette was 94 per cent and the smallest proportion 47 per cent. Indeed, in only one case (Vignette 6) were there more informants who did not include assessment in their discussion than those who did. Chi-square analysis reveals that in five cases out of seven the difference between recognition and non-recognition was statistically significant. Thus it seems that

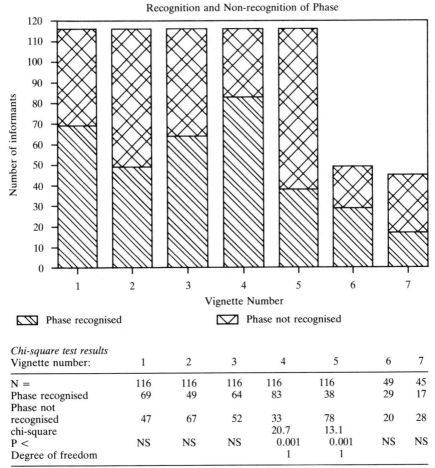

Number of informants (y-axis)

Recognition and Non-recognition of Phase

Vignette Number

☒ Phase recognised   ☒ Phase not recognised

Chi-square test results

Vignette number:	1	2	3	4	5	6	7
N =	116	116	116	116	116	49	45
Phase recognised	69	49	64	83	38	29	17
Phase not recognised	47	67	52	33	78	20	28
chi-square				20.7	13.1		
P <	NS	NS	NS	0.001	0.001	NS	NS
Degree of freedom				1	1		

Critical values of chi-square (two tailed) at one degree of freedom = 3.84 (0.05), 6.64 (0.01), 10.83 (0.001).

Figure 6.1   Problem identification

problem assessment is generally well recognised, and better recognised than problem identification. There is little doubt that problem assessment is a significant step in nursing problem solving.

The assessment phase in Vignettes 2 and 3 was deliberately omitted, but interestingly, in both cases the majority of informants either recognised this omission or continued to discuss this phase as if it had been included. In only one of these two cases, however, (Vignette 3) was the difference between recognition and non-recognition statistically significant.

The majority of informants also failed to discuss assessment in Vignette

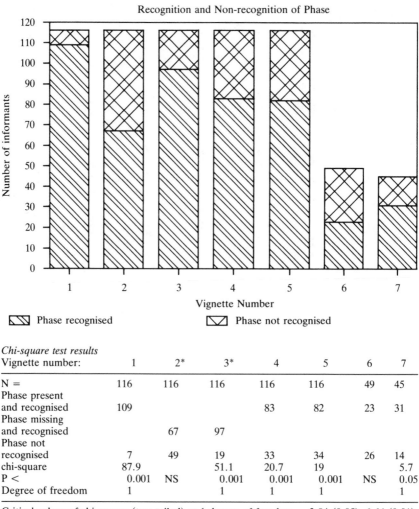

Figure 6.2 Problem assessment

6, but the difference between recognition and non-recognition was not statistically significant.

It is hard to explain this result, particularly when Vignette 6 included an explicit account of the assessment phase, but the sample was smaller here than with the other vignettes.

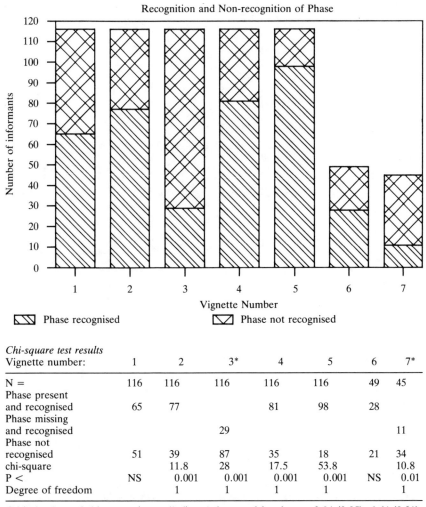

Figure 6.3 shows Recognition and Non-recognition of Phase

Figure 6.3 Planning

Chi-square test results

Vignette number:	1	2	3*	4	5	6	7*
N =	116	116	116	116	116	49	45
Phase present and recognised	65	77		81	98	28	
Phase missing and recognised			29				11
Phase not recognised	51	39	87	35	18	21	34
chi-square		11.8	28	17.5	53.8		10.8
P <	NS	0.001	0.001	0.001	0.001	NS	0.01
Degree of freedom		1	1	1	1		1

Critical values of chi-square (two-tailed) at 1 degree of freedom = 3.84 (0.05), 6.64 (0.01), 10.83 (0.001).
* Planning deliberately omitted from this vignette.

3. Planning

Figure 6.3 shows that in Vignettes 2, 4 and 5 (where the planning phase was made explicit) the majority of informants recognised this phase, and in every case the difference between recognition and non-recognition was statistically significant. On the other hand, Vignettes 1 and 6 also included

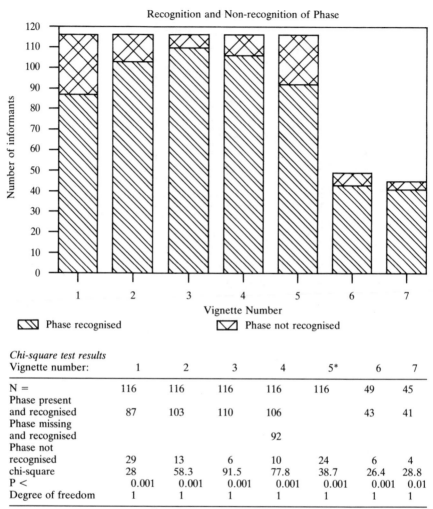

Recognition and Non-recognition of Phase

Phase recognised   Phase not recognised

Chi-square test results

Vignette number:	1	2	3	4	5*	6	7
N =	116	116	116	116	116	49	45
Phase present and recognised	87	103	110	106		43	41
Phase missing and recognised					92		
Phase not recognised	29	13	6	10	24	6	4
chi-square	28	58.3	91.5	77.8	38.7	26.4	28.8
P <	0.001	0.001	0.001	0.001	0.001	0.001	0.01
Degree of freedom	1	1	1	1	1	1	1

Critical values of chi-square (two-tailed) at 1 degree of freedom = 3.84 (0.05), 6.64 (0.01), 10.83 (0.001).
* Implementation deliberately omitted from this vignette.

Figure 6.4 Implementation

an explanation of the planning phase, but the differences here were not statistically significant.

In the vignettes where planning had been omitted (Vignettes 3 and 7), the majority of the sample failed to recognise this omission. In both cases the difference between non-recognition and recognition was statistically significant. In total, 55 per cent of informants commented on planning – not as high a proportion as might be expected.

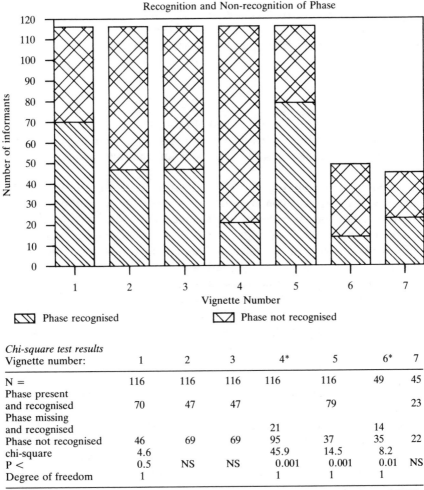

Chi-square test results

Vignette number:	1	2	3	4*	5	6*	7
N =	116	116	116	116	116	49	45
Phase present and recognised	70	47	47		79		23
Phase missing and recognised				21		14	
Phase not recognised	46	69	69	95	37	35	22
chi-square	4.6			45.9	14.5	8.2	
P <	0.5	NS	NS	0.001	0.001	0.01	NS
Degree of freedom	1			1	1	1	

Critical values of chi-square (two-tailed) at 1 degree of freedom = 3.84 (0.05), 6.64 (0.01), 10.83 (0.001)
* Evaluation deliberately omitted from this vignette.

Figure 6.5 Evaluation

4. Implementation

The number of comments on implementation well outnumbered comments on its nearest rival (assessment). Eighty-seven per cent of the informants commented on implementation, and this phase shows the greatest consistency in the frequency of recognition and non-recognition (Figure 6.4). In all seven vignettes the majority of informants discussed implementation, including Vignette 5 in which this phase was omitted. The difference between those who recognised the phase and those who failed to comment was statistically significant in each case. Clearly, implementation should be regarded as a particularly important phase in nursing problem-solving.

5. Evaluation

This last element in the phase model of problem-solving attracted far less attention than problem identification, assessment, planning and implementation. In total, only 44 per cent of the informants discussed evaluation.

As can be seen from Figure 6.5, in only three of the seven cases did the majority of informants comment on this phase. However, in only two of these was the difference statistically significant.

On the other hand, in Vignettes 2, 3, 4 and 6, only a minority of informants commented on evaluation, but in only two of these cases where the phase was deliberately omitted was the difference between non-recognition and recognition statistically significant. The lack of attention devoted to evaluation by nurses in this study is surprising in view of the attention given to this stage in both the general problem-solving literature (see Table 2.2) and the specific literature relating to nursing. This issue is discussed further in Chapters 7 and 8.

Informants' pathway through vignettes

One interesting finding arising out of the qualitative analysis was that when informants discussed phases they did not necessarily do so sequentially. Typically, individuals explored the vignettes non-linearly, and often began their discussion at the second, third or fourth phase, rather than starting at problem identification and progressing through assessment, planning, implementation and evaluation.

It was decided, therefore, to examine this finding in more detail. Figure 6.6 shows a nurse manager's pathway through Vignettes 1, 2 and 3, based on an analysis of the transcript of the informant's interview.

The coding of transcripts and the validation of the coding system is described above (pp. 52–57).

In Figure 6.6, there does not appear to be a pattern of comment, except the informant's repeated discussion of implementation in Vignette 2. When this analysis is extended to other transcripts (see Appendix 5) it is found that there is no similarity between any one informant's pathway and that of another. The one recurrent feature was the informants' habit of returning to problem identification and even more so to implementation,

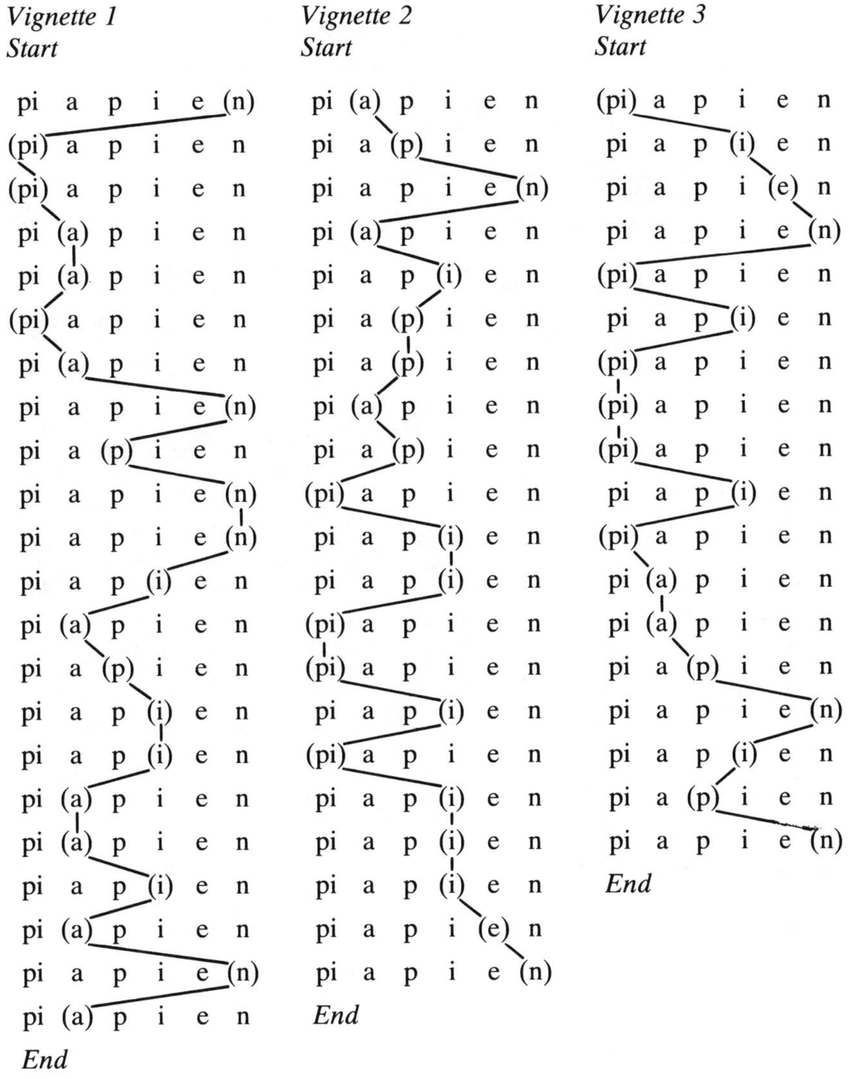

Vignette 1	Vignette 2	Vignette 3
Start	*Start*	*Start*

```
Vignette 1          Vignette 2          Vignette 3
Start               Start               Start

pi  a  p  i  e (n)  pi (a) p  i  e  n  (pi) a  p  i  e  n
(pi) a  p  i  e  n  pi  a (p) i  e  n  pi  a  p (i) e  n
(pi) a  p  i  e  n  pi  a  p  i  e (n) pi  a  p  i (e) n
pi (a) p  i  e  n   pi (a) p  i  e  n  pi  a  p  i  e (n)
pi (a) p  i  e  n   pi  a  p (i) e  n  (pi) a  p  i  e  n
(pi) a  p  i  e  n  pi  a (p) i  e  n  pi  a  p (i) e  n
pi (a) p  i  e  n   pi  a (p) i  e  n  (pi) a  p  i  e  n
pi  a  p  i  e (n)  pi (a) p  i  e  n  (pi) a  p  i  e  n
pi  a (p) i  e  n   pi  a (p) i  e  n  (pi) a  p  i  e  n
pi  a  p  i  e (n)  (pi) a  p  i  e  n pi  a  p (i) e  n
pi  a  p  i  e (n)  pi  a  p (i) e  n  (pi) a  p  i  e  n
pi  a  p (i) e  n   pi  a  p (i) e  n  pi (a) p  i  e  n
pi (a) p  i  e  n   (pi) a  p  i  e  n pi (a) p  i  e  n
pi  a (p) i  e  n   (pi) a  p  i  e  n pi  a (p) i  e  n
pi  a  p (i) e  n   pi  a  p (i) e  n  pi  a  p  i  e (n)
pi  a  p (i) e  n   (pi) a  p  i  e  n pi  a  p (i) e  n
pi (a) p  i  e  n   pi  a  p (i) e  n  pi  a (p) i  e  n
pi (a) p  i  e  n   pi  a  p (i) e  n  pi  a  p  i  e (n)
pi  a  p (i) e  n   pi  a  p (i) e  n  End
pi (a) p  i  e  n   pi  a  p  i (e) n
pi  a  p  i  e (n)  pi  a  p  i  e (n)
pi (a) p  i  e  n   End
End
```

Key:
Problem identification	(pi)
Assessment	(a)
Planning	(p)
Implementation	(i)
Evaluation	(e)
Not definable	(n)

Figure 6.6 One informant's pathway through Vignettes 1, 2 and 3

Problem-solving in Nursing Practice

Table 6.2 Recognition and non-recognition of phases by informants with different levels of experience (N = 116)

Key: a phase present, and presence recognised
    b phase present but no comment made
    c phase missing, and omission recognised
    d phase missing but no comment made
    * Including learner nurses who are categorised as zero
 ₁ ** Critical value of chi-square at 2 degrees of freedom = 4.6 (0.10), 5.99 (0.05), 9.21 (0.01)

	Identif.		Assess.		Plann.		Implem.		Evaluat.	
Vignette 1	a	b	a	b	a	b	a	b	a	b
0–2.11 yrs*	17	17	32	2	14	20	30	4	20	14
3–5.11 yrs	23	10	29	4	16	17	21	12	24	9
6+ yrs	29	20	48	1	35	14	36	13	26	23
chi-square	2.7		3.54		8.52**		5.51		3.23	
P	NS		NS		<0.05		<0.10		NS	
Vignette 2	a	b	c	d	a	b	a	b	a	b
0–2.11 yrs*	15	19	17	17	22	12	32	2	15	19
3–5.11 yrs	16	17	23	10	22	11	26	7	12	21
6+ yrs	28	21	27	22	33	16	45	4	20	29
chi-square	1.47		2.91		0.06		4.75		0.42	
P	NS		NS		NS		<0.10		NS	
Vignette 3	a	b	c	d	c	d	a	b	a	b
0–2.11 yrs*	14	20	23	11	8	26	32	1	17	17
3–5.11 yrs	23	10	30	3	8	25	32	1	14	18
6+ yrs	27	22	44	5	13	36	46	3	16	33
chi-square	5.51		8.98**		5.51		0.02		2.65	
P	<0.10		<0.05		<0.10		NS		NS	
Vignette 4	a	b	a	b	a	b	a	b	c	d
0–2.11 yrs*	18	16	25	9	21	13	32	2	2	32
3–5.11 yrs	24	9	23	10	23	10	28	5	10	23
6+ yrs	31	18	35	14	37	12	46	3	9	40
chi-square	2.81		0.12		1.8		0.54		6.74**	
P	NS		NS		NS		NS		<0.05	
Vignette 5	a	b	a	b	a	b	c	d	a	b
0–2.11 yrs*	6	28	19	15	27	7	27	7	26	8
3–5.11 yrs	13	20	25	8	29	4	24	9	19	14
6+ yrs	19	30	38	11	42	7	41	8	34	15
chi-square	4.99		5.12		1.01		1.44		2.82	
P	<0.10		<0.10		NS		NS		NS	
Vignette 6	a	b	a	b	a	b	a	b	c	d
0–2.11 yrs*	13	6	8	11	12	7	19	0	7	12
3–5.11 yrs	6	8	9	5	5	8	11	3	4	10
6+ yrs	10	6	6	10	11	5	13	3	3	13
chi-square	2.29		2.44		3.01		4.38		1.39	
P	NS		NS		NS		NS		NS	
Vignette 7	a	b	a	b	c	d	a	b	a	b
0–2.11 yrs*	3	11	11	3	2	12	14	0	9	5
3–5.11 yrs	4	8	4	8	3	9	11	1	7	5
6+ yrs	10	9	16	3	6	13	16	3	7	12
chi-square	2.29		9.77**		1.31		2.49		2.77	
P	NS		<0.01		NS		NS		NS	

which confirms the notion that nurses are concerned with the 'doing' aspect of nursing problem-solving. Indeed, informants may have concentrated on implementation at the expense of the other phases. But it must be remembered that nurses are commenting on second-hand problem scenarios, and there is no guarantee that they would follow the same thought processes in real problem-solving situations.

Nurses' problem-solving at different levels of experience

Following a preliminary analysis of the transcripts, it appeared that the more experienced nurses had a deeper perception of clinical problem-solving and recognised missing phases more consistently.

To explore this issue further, the recognition and non-recognition of phases by nurses with different levels of experience were compared. Table 6.2 presents a summary of this analysis.

Nurses' experience was categorised in three ways. First, nurses with up to three years' experience (including learner nurses) were classified as the 'least experienced' group. Second, nurses with between three and six years' experience were classified as the 'middle experienced' group. And third, nurses with more than six years' experience were classified as the 'most experienced' group. It is clear from Table 6.2 that the researcher's initial impression of differences in perception between nurses with different experiences was not supported.

When these data were compared using the chi-square test, in only 4 of 35 cases were the differences statistically significant. Even then no pattern emerges. In summary:

Groups of Data with a Significant Statistical Difference of P <0.05 or P <0.01

Vignette 1 (patient with insomia): Planning
The 'most experienced' nurses commented more on the use of planning than the 'less experienced' and the 'middle experienced' groups.

Vignette 3 (parents who complained): Assessment
Assessment was recognised as missing by the majority of informants in all groups. The 'most experienced' and the 'middle experienced' group of nurses, however, commented more on this phase.

Vignette 4 (patient who has undergone enucleation): Evaluation
Here, the order is reversed. Rather surprisingly, the majority of informants in all groups failed to recognise that evaluation was missing. However, more of the 'middle experienced' informants recognised the omission.

Vignette 7 (patient with diabetes): Assessment
Here, more of the informants from the 'least experienced' and 'most experienced' groups recognised this phase. However, not too much emphasis should be placed on this finding because of the small cell sizes.

Owing both to the small number of statistically significant findings and to the absence of any pattern in the data, it appears that recognition and non-recognition of problem-solving phases is not strongly dependent on experience.

This chapter has presented an overview of nurses' perceptions of clinical problem-solving. This quantitative analysis should be seen in the context of the qualitative analysis which follows in the next chapter, where some of the issues raised here are discussed in more detail.

7

Qualitative Analysis of the Transcripts

A qualitative analysis of the interview transcripts was undertaken to illuminate nursing problem-solving further. In most cases, the analysis reinforces the findings discussed in Chapter 6, but some new and important issues are raised, which to date have attracted little comment in the literature.

The analysis resulted in the identification of 51 categories of response. As discussed above (p. 54), a particular category was identified when at least five informants freely commented about the issue(s). The categories are listed in Table 7.1 and subsumed under the five phases of problem-solving.

Table 7.1 shows some interesting variations in the responses from the different types of nurse.

Learner nurses were included in the study in order to compare their perceptions of problem-solving with those of more experienced nurses, and it is significant that learner nurses were generally well represented in almost all categories. This was an unexpected finding in view of some statements in the nursing literature about the relationship between poor problem-solving and inexperience (see McCarthy, 1981; Corcoran, 1986). Indeed, the proportion of learner nurses who commented on an important facet of problem-solving sometimes exceeded the proportion of any other category of nurse (see Table 7.1, Categories: 11, 14, 28, 29, 31, 32, 42 and 47). One reason for these differences may be that learner nurses are well practised in reflecting on case study materials through recent training.

At the other extreme, in terms of experience, nurse managers, although somewhat divorced from day-to-day nursing, were not particularly distinguishable from other categories of nurse in their choice of response. These findings are in line with the results of the statistical analysis on the degree of recognition and non-recognition of phases by informants with different levels of experience (Table 6.2).

Table 7.1 The type and proportion of informants who discussed a category of response

Key: L = learner nurse
      S = staff nurse
      W = ward sister/charge nurse
      T = nurse teacher
      M = nurse manager

Category of response	Proportion of informants (%)					
	L	S	W	T	M	Total
N =	22	17	44	21	12	116
Problem identification	%	%	%	%	%	%
1. Summarising and clarifying the problem	41	41	36	81	25	45
2. Classifying the problem	14	0	9	19	17	11
3. Overlooked important problems and sub-problems	9	18	9	0	0	8
4. Identifying problems and sub-problems	27	29	70	62	67	54
5. Prioritising problems	18	0	7	14	17	10
6. Confirming the problem	23	53	52	33	42	42
7. Timing of problem identification	45	35	43	24	25	37
Problem assessment						
8. Summarising assessment data	82	53	55	71	58	63
9. Quality judgements in assessment	59	35	48	33	42	45
10. Seeking additional assessment data	18	24	34	24	50	29
11. Sources of assessment information	86	29	80	71	75	72
12. Confirming assessment data	36	18	34	10	25	27
13. Timing of assessment	68	47	70	52	92	66
14. Identifying problems and sub-problems from assessment	86	47	66	86	58	70
15. The most appropriate assessor	9	12	0	5	25	7
16. Assessment skills	18	12	25	19	25	21
17. Two-stage and multi-stage assessment	36	18	14	5	58	22
Planning						
18. Relationship between planning and assessment	23	12	23	24	42	23
19. Summarising the plan	9	24	27	33	8	22
20. Quality judgements in planning	50	24	43	33	50	41
21. The problem component	14	18	20	14	25	18
22. The goal component	77	76	75	76	75	76
23. The intervention component	45	0	32	48	17	31
24. Role of patient and others	59	41	52	71	58	56
25. Nursing experience in planning	5	6	9	14	8	9
26. Place of medical treatment	9	12	14	10	8	11
Implementation						
27. Summarising implementation	68	24	55	52	50	52
28. Judging the quality of implementation	100	47	59	76	58	68
29. Alternative and/or additional interventions	86	53	55	71	75	66

Category of response	Proportion of informants (%)					
30. Timing and sequencing of interventions	68	35	55	57	75	57
31. Role of patient, relative, and ex-patient	73	47	59	57	42	58
32. Role of other health workers	68	41	50	48	50	52
33. Role of planning/goals	27	18	50	43	25	37
34. Role of the problem	5	35	27	19	0	20
35. Role of assessment	14	12	16	24	25	17
36. Role of ward routine	14	0	9	0	0	6
37. Educational value of implementation for learners	43	35	30	38	33	35
38. Recording nursing interventions	41	24	25	38	25	30
Evaluation						
39. Summarising evaluation	36	18	32	29	33	30
40. Quality judgements in evaluation	18	12	18	10	8	15
41. Assessment as a synonym for evaluation	9	6	7	0	8	6
42. Evaluation issues	82	41	52	62	33	56
43. Frequency of evaluation	45	24	25	33	25	30
44. Role of nurse and other health workers	32	12	7	33	42	21
45. Role of patient, parent and family	18	6	14	29	0	15
46. A means of determining patient's progress	23	12	18	10	0	15
47. A means of judging the plan or action	59	47	43	38	33	45
48. A means of identifying new problems	14	12	9	10	8	10
49. Assessment following evaluation	9	0	7	19	8	9
50. Evaluation in the sequence of problem solving	5	0	2	14	8	5
51. Recording and communicating evaluation evidence	9	18	5	10	0	8

Each category of response will now be discussed and illustrated with quotations from the transcripts. Because of the way responses were categorised, it was felt that statistical analysis was not justified.

1. Problem identification

This phase attracted the lowest number of comments (238) of all the five phases. However, seven categories of response emerge following an analysis of informants' discussion of problem identification during the course of the interviews.

1. Summarising and clarifying the problem

Informants (particularly a high proportion of nurse teachers) often began their discussion by simply summarising the problem statement in the vignette. Others rephrased and reinterpreted the scenario for themselves using words with which they felt more comfortable.

The first illustration of this category is a quotation from a learner nurse discussing Vignette 6 (patient with a circulatory problem). The next two extracts, from interviews with more experienced nurses, show similar reinterpretations. The second quotation came from a staff nurse discussing Vignette 3 (parents who complained) and the third from a nurse teacher discussing Vignette 7 (patient with diabetes):

> 'This problem is about orthopaedic surgery and a patient with an unattended arm. Sister is going round checking him three hours after theatre. Possibly other nurses are attending to the patient, but if they are, they haven't picked up the circulatory problem. But even if they haven't, sister should have seen it before.'

> 'The parents are complaining about their child's care when they seem most uncaring parents themselves. The father is a business executive, which seems to be priority number one, and his wife seems to care more for her mother, which isn't a bad thing, but when you have an ill daughter the baby ought to come first.'

> 'I think the nursing actions stem from the fact that he is a 45-year-old school teacher happily married with two teenage children and that no one in the family has suffered any serious illness before. Now he has diabetes and feels unable to cope.'

2. Classifying the problem

Another interpretive activity was to clarify the problem in some way. Occasionally, the identified problems were divided into the main or sub-problems. Some informants were quick to point out that problems were either medical or nursing. The most popular way of classifying problems, however, was to use the term 'actual' or 'potential' problem, as shown in this comment from a manager discussing Vignette 1 (patient with insomnia):

> 'Sister should have had this problem noted as a potential problem'.

Summarising, clarifying and classifying problems appeared to be ways in which informants focused on the patient's needs.

3. Overlooked important problems and sub-problems

Informants sometimes added problems to those discussed in the vignettes if it was felt that important problems had been left out. Two reasons why problems might be overlooked are illustrated by a comment from a charge nurse discussing Vignette 1 (patient with insomnia), and by a sister who commented on Vignette 3 (parents who complained):

'I was interested in this one from the point of view that the sister used a clear, logical approach. I think a systematic approach to problem-solving is important, but I would like to add that an adherence to a strict, rigid code of organisation can lead you up the wrong avenue, which prevents you from finding out what the patient's main or other problems might be.'

'The sister was on the defensive, caught off-guard, and she didn't recognise the true problem. Her solution, therefore was inapproproate.'

4. Identifying problems and sub-problems

Almost half of the informants (generally experienced staff) discussed how the problem was brought to the nurse's attention. Most felt it was appropriate that the patient should tell the nurse of a problem. It was further pointed out that a nurse should be careful how he or she articulates a problem in case problems were suggested to the patient. The quotation below is an example of this latter issue, and was made by a sister commenting on Vignette 1 (patient with insomnia):

'Perhaps the sister should not have suggested work as being a problem to the patient. It would have been better to ask the patient if there were any more problems.'

Instances that appeared to cause concern and possibly embarrassment were those where the nurse was told of a nursing problem by a relative or a doctor, rather than finding the problem herself. The following comment from a learner nurse discussing Vignette 4 (patient who has undergone enucleation) highlights this:

'I mean, you have to question that it is the mother who observes the change and reports the problem to the ward sister and not the nursing staff who spot the problem.'

Some informants commented on the issue of problems being recognised by learner nurses. In such cases it was emphasised (by the more experienced nurses) that inexperienced nurses should always report the problem to the ward manager so that it could be dealt with effectively. It was suggested, however, that the nurse in charge should include the learner nurse in subsequent actions.

Some informants felt that the problem had been identified incorrectly. This error, it was suggested, led to focusing incorrectly on the patient's nursing requirments. As one nurse manager (discussing Vignette 4, patient who has undergone enucleation) explained:

'She says that withdrawal is the main problem, but I think angry might be a better description. They also seem to be making a fuss about his physical appearance which might not be his problem and might be making it into a problem even though he didn't have one. So it could be problem causing rather than problem identifying.'

The last quotation also suggests that some of the problems described in the vignettes were created needlessly. It was felt that some problems should be considered normal for that situation and that, as one nurse tutor said: 'it is easy to become problem-oriented' with the approaches used by the nurses in the vignettes.

5. Prioritising problems

Stating problems in order of importance was mentioned by a few informants (12). For example, a learner nurse commenting on Vignette 5 (patient with angina) explained:

> 'Mrs Forest's main problem is her anxiety because two members of her family have already died of the same sort of thing. Smoking and obesity are secondary problems . . .'

Some informants felt that in at least one vignette the patients' problems had been prioritised incorrectly, with the more serious problems being deferred until the end. Several reasons were suggested for this. One was that the nurse lacked knowledge of and experience with particularly difficult problems; another suggested reason was the lack of commitment to problem-solving by some nurses.

6. Confirming the problem

Informants were equally divided on whether the identified problem should or should not be confirmed with evidence from another source. One group said that problems identified by a nurse, patient or relative should not be taken at face-value by the ward manager. The problem should, wherever possible, be confirmed by another nurse, by the patient (frequently mentioned) or by a doctor, using, if appropriate, more objective data such as a laboratory report. It was felt in particular that problems identified by learner nurses should be followed up in this way. Two quotations which highlight the issue of confirming the problem are given below. The first came from a sister discussing Vignette 1 (patient with insomnia), and the second from a sister discussing Vignette 2 (patient with an inflamed wound):

> 'I liked the way the sister went to interview the patient. She didn't just accept the night nurse's word. She also looked to see if it had been documented as a problem.'

> 'The learner nurse identified the problem and the sister planned the care. Was there in fact a problem? The sister hasn't yet looked at the wound and determined if the problem exists.'

There were, however, an equal number of informants who felt that nurses should *not* seek corroborative evidence and that the patient should be trusted. Some expressed surprise and disbelief that nurses sought supportive evidence. The quotations below illustrate how the informant is prepared to trust the patient's view. The first came from a nurse teacher and the second from a sister, both discussing Vignette 1 (patient with insomnia):

> 'I know that patients often tell the nurse that they haven't slept a wink all night, when they have been fast asleep, but even so it's nice to think that a nurse would have a little more trust in patients.'

> 'If the patient says they are in pain, or have a problem, well that is the way it is. It may be just the way the problem is worded, but to confirm that the problem exists is just wrong.'

The majority of comments on confirming the problem came from the more experienced nurses.

7. Timing of problem identification

This category was discussed by almost half the learner nurses and ward sisters. Some said that the patient's problem must be identified as early as possible; see for example the comment below from a learner nurse discussing Vignette 6 (patient with a circulatory problem):

> 'I will tell you one thing, the patient's fingers are blue, cold and tingling. This should have been found much quicker because of the danger of stopping his circulation. It takes quite a while for this to happen.'

The issue of timing was also evident in this comment from a nurse manager discussing Vignette 4 (patient who has undergone enucleation):

> 'The main thing about this is that the problem . . . could have been avoided. It was solved after the event, rather than something which could have been seen before it caused the patient to be unhappy.'

There was concern that the patient's recovery would be delayed, or that he or she might even be harmed if the problem was identified too late. Some felt that the whole care situation was jeopardised because of the delay, a view clearly expressed in the quotation below which came from a sister discussing Vignette 4 (patient who has undergone enucleation):

> 'What I particularly disliked about this was that he is nearly ready for discharge and then they discover that he is withdrawn. It seems to me that they might have sent him home when he was feeling suicidal. Thank heaven his mother pointed this out.'

It was suggested that one way of minimising these difficulties was to individualise patient care by assigning one or more nurses to a patient.

Finally, informants' discussion of problem identification often merged with their comments on problem assessment. Also, despite the fact that problem identification was explicit and appeared first within each vignette, it was not always considered first (Figure 6.6). For example, informants sometimes discussed problems after they had examined the way the assessment had been done. Bearing these two points in mind there is some doubt from this research that problem identification can always be regarded as an initial and distinct phase in clinical problem-solving, even though it is one of the most frequently cited stages in the problem-solving literature (see Table 2.2).

One possible explanation for the merger of problem identification with assessment is that the nursing records used by many Districts reflect the nursing process. The records (an example of which is set out below) do not include problem identification as a separate phase and this practice may have influenced informants' thinking. A typical record, used in a District from which part of the sample was taken, has the following components:

1. nursing assessment and statement of nursing problems;
2. nursing plan, including the problem statement and goals;
3. nursing interventions made;
4. evaluation of patient's progress.*

Problem identification and consequently problem statement are implicit within the assessment and planning phases.

Summary of the problem identification phase

The findings from the qualitative analysis of this phase are summarised by listing the points that support statements in the literature and those on which there is less or no particular support in the literature.

The views and statements on problem identification in this study support the literature as follows:

1. problems and sub-problems are usually classified in some way (Roper et al., 1983, p. 10);
2. problems can be identified from many sources and by several means (Johnson et al., 1980, pp. 47–57);
3. timing of problem identification is felt to be crucial to the patient's well-being (Bailey and Claus, 1975, p. 21: Yeaw, 1979).

* Source: Nursing process documents from Central Nottinghamshire Health Authority, 1987.

Notably, this research has revealed an issue of problem identification not usually discussed in the literature, namely, problems should be confirmed, especially when an inexperienced nurse is the source.

2. Problem assessment

Next to implementation, assessment was the phase which attracted the most comment from informants. Consequently, ten categories of response emerge from an analysis of the transcripts.

8. Summarising assessment data

A large proportion (63 per cent) of the informants summarised the description of assessment in the vignettes. This seemed to be one way informants focused on the individual problem and tended to occur even when the assessment phase was deliberately missing from the vignette. Two examples of summarising are given below. The first is a comment made by a staff nurse discussing Vignette 5 (patient with angina) and the second from a nurse teacher summarising Vignette 7 (patient with diabetes):

'Although the patient is happily married, she admits to being a worrier. This is somebody who has stress in her life. Also, she has a job which might be classed as stress-causing. She also smokes. These are all known factors attributed to heart disease.'

'She [the sister] takes a look at the social and economic background to this gentleman. He is a 45-year-old school teacher, happily married with teenage children. This is as much as she needs to know about this chap. She has sat down and talked to him about his condition, so she has gone through a process of factual assessment for want of a better word.'

The description of the assessment given in Vignettes 1, 4, 5, 6 and 7 (assessment had been omitted from 2 and 3), was necessarily brief to keep the vignettes within the prescribed length (see p. 47). It is perhaps not surprising, therefore, that informants interpreted the information provided to their own satisfaction to facilitate discussion. Two extracts from interview transcripts which emphasise this point are given below. The first came from a nurse teacher discussing Vignette 4 (patient who has undergone enucleation) and the second was a comment made by a charge nurse discussing Vignette 3 (parents who complained), one which did not include assessment:

'A guy of 19 who has lost an eye is going to be worried about his sexuality. It must be devastating to have your appearance altered in this way with your whole life still in front of you. It must make him feel low just to think of it. I think he is heading for almost a clinical depression.'

'I just wonder if the outburst has arisen because the mother is under a lot of stress at home. Was it because she is too busy looking after her own mother without the support of her husband? I get the feeling there are many more family problems here, more than what is coming out. It could also be the result of the parent's guilt; skeletons in the cupboard we don't know about.'

Embellishment of the vignettes, as in these quotations, was particularly noticeable in the interviews with expert informants. For example, an orthopaedic nurse teacher discussing Vignette 6 (patient with a circulatory problem) said:

'Although I do feel that the circulatory problem is caused by the tight plaster, it did cross my mind that there might be something more seriously wrong. There is a complication of this type of surgery called Compartment Syndrome, I would wonder at the time of the assessment if that was happening.'

From these and other comments, it would seem that the degree of interpretation of the assessment information reflects the extent of the informant's experience.

9.   Quality judgements in assessment

Nearly half (45 per cent) of the informants commented on the quality of the assessment process and/or the resultant data. These 'process' and 'outcome' issues are highlighted in the comments below. In the first quotation a sister, discussing Vignette 1 (patient with insomnia), commented on the consequences of the nurse's initial poor assessment. And in the second a nurse manager praised the assessment process in Vignette 7 (patient with diabetes):

'The assessment was superficial. All the factors were not considered, hence the need to assess again following the poor resolution . . .'

'I think that the sister is excellent in the way she discovered why he can't give his own insulin because he can't accept his illness . . .'

Some went on to suggest further action, an issue discussed in the category that follows.

10.   Seeking additional assessment data

Informants sometimes recommended that additional data would need to be collected. Indeed, some felt strongly that there were insufficient data in the vignettes and went on to suggest what else was required. This is illustrated in the following statement from a sister discussing the need to examine diet in Vignette 7 (patient with diabetes):

'Once again we need more information. We need to go on to food and the
changes in his diet because of the diabetes. It's useful to find out what his
food likes and dislikes are . . .'

11. Sources of assessment information

Many ways and means of collecting data were mentioned during the
interviews, and sources of information were commonly discussed by all
groups except staff nurses. A charge nurse, for example, discussing
Vignette 1 (patient with insomnia) explained one source:

'This assessment included the patient's perceptions of the problem, for the
patient is asked to explain her usual sleeping pattern.'

Examples of patient-specific sources of further information, as suggested
by informants (many of these sources can be expected to feature in the
patient's nursing records), are listed below:

1. an investigation of the patient's clinical features;
2. the patient's performance in one or more activities of living (cf. Roper
   et al., 1983);
3. the patient's perception of the problem;
4. the patient and problem in relation to family, job, financial status, and
   friends, etc.;
5. the effect of related problems;
6. the problem in relation to the lapse of time between the present and
   last nursing intervention;
7. the results of some nursing or medical measure; for example, the
   patient's temperature, or wound swab results;
8. the patient's immediate or long-term needs; for example, the effects of
   the problem on his or her ability to walk.

In addition to these, informants also suggested the following sources of
information:

1. parents of young patients;
2. family member, relative or friend;
3. nurses who are involved in the patient's care;
4. patient's doctor;
5. other health-care workers involved in the care;
6. community staff;
7. social services officer;
8. patient's employer;
9. other patients.

Considering the extent to which nursing models have been written and
talked about generally in nursing articles prior to and during the data

collection phase of this research, it is surprising that models did not feature more strongly in the informants' discussion of the assessment phase. From 116 interviews, only two informants (both nurse teachers) suggested the nurse should base an assessment on a nursing model. The two models mentioned were (1) the 'model of living' described by Roper et al. (1983); and (2) the Roy adaptation model (Riehl and Roy, 1980). References to the models were brief, for example, a nurse teacher discussing Vignette 1 (patient with insomnia) said:

> 'I don't know which model the sister has used when she was looking at the patient, but it looks very much like a Roy adaptation model; looking at the environment and what have you . . . because it looked at the environment it would fit in very well with the contextual and residual stimuli. It would all fit in very nicely. The first-stage assessment is where you look at all the physical, psychological, and sociological things. It looks at self-concepts, interdependence, help-seeking and others . . .'

It may be that models are still considered to be a new concept in nursing and have not yet been fully assimilated into nursing practice.

12.   Confirming assessment data

As in the case of problem identification, some informants (27 per cent – proportionally more learner nurses and sisters) said there was a need to corroborate findings from one assessment with evidence from another source. But fewer informants commented on the confirmation of assessment data compared with problem identification (42 per cent). An example of corroboration of assessment data follows where a nurse teacher discussed the reliabilty of the patient's information in Vignette 6 (patient with a circulatory problem) said:

> 'When sister examines the patient's arm and questions him about it she discovers some important facts. It says that he is sleepy, so I don't think she should have taken that as part of her assessment really, because the patient was quite drowsy, although he was talking to other patients. I still don't think he would have been a reliable source. She should have physically checked his sensation and circulation as well as asking the patient about them.'

The reader may recall from Category 6 (p. 76) (confirming the problem) that some informants objected to the principle of seeking corroborative evidence, and that the patient should be trusted. But there were no such dissenters in the case of assessment; for example, no one said it was unprofessional to check an issue a patient claimed to be relevant to the problem.

It was generally felt to be important that a more experienced nurse should confirm the assessment data provided by a learner nurse. In addition, it was suggested that the experienced nurse should be accompanied by a learner nurse when carrying out an assessment. When questioned about this, informants explained that the learner nurse would benefit from the experience and probably make a contribution by adding other perceptions.

If the nurse believed that a problem might lead to a complaint or other untoward incident, it was recommended that a second nurse witness the assessment. It was recognised, however, that this was not always feasible. As one charge nurse explained, 'it is not always possible to triangulate during an assessment . . .'

13. Timing of assessment

The most appropriate time for assessing was frequently discussed, particularly by a high proportion (92 per cent) of the nurse managers. The two extracts below, typical of this category, illustrate the importance of timing. The first comment was made by a nurse manager discussing Vignette 1 (patient with insomnia), and the second by a staff nurse discussing Vignette 3 (parents who complained):

> 'I can't believe that the assessment was done after the problem came to light! The sister should have assessed fully on admission and the problems and potential problems identified.'

> 'It is a pity that this incident occurred in the first place. The ward staff should have been aware at assessment that problems might occur, because the parents would not be able to stay with their child and so could not participate more fully in her care.'

As discussed earlier in this chapter (see Category 7, timing of problem identification), it was not always clear from the discussion that nurses made a crisp distinction between problem identification and assessment. Some informants felt that the nurse should assess the patient on admission to identify the problems (as in the first quotation above), while others said that these should be listed and used to structure the assessment.

The place of assessment in relation to the remaining phases was discussed from other perspectives too. For example, it was pointed out the nursing plan, or nursing intervention, would be inappropriate if it were not based on an assessment. In the first quotation below a learner nurse, discussing Vignette 3 (parents who complained), criticised the ward sister's actions. In the second example, a sister discussing Vignette 2 (patient with an inflamed wound) also questioned the sister's actions:

> 'Whilst I agree the sister should apologise to the parents, but to reassure them that this will definitely not happen again is crazy. She didn't even know what happened in the first place, the nappy might have been changed recently, she didn't check this. It isn't a good excuse either to say that the

ward is busy. The parents won't particularly care about that even though it might be true.'

'Well, she just took the learner's word for it. The learner might have been very inexperienced. The sister should have gone and assessed the wound before she set those goals. In any case, it would have been an ideal learning opportunity for the student.'

Some informants suggested a form of nursing intervention, such as reassuring the patient, coming between a two-stage assessment. This can be seen in the following extract from an interview with a sister discussing Vignette 1 (patient with insomnia):

'There wasn't enough explanation given to the patient. She is bound to be anxious about her headaches. Reassurance could have been given at the time of the assessment which would have helped the sister to get more information out of the patient.'

It would appear that the timing of assessment is a complex issue, which depends on the context of the problem and the skill and experience of the assessor, points which are further discussed under Category 15 (the most appropriate assessor) and Category 16 (assessment skills) to follow.

14. Identifying problems and sub-problems from assessment

Many informants felt strongly that one of the functions of assessment was to identify related problems. As can be seen from Table 7.1, this category attracted a lot of comment, particularly a high proportion of learner nurses (86 per cent) and nurse teachers (86 per cent).

In the first and second quotations below a charge nurse and staff nurse, respectively, discuss this issue when commenting on Vignette 1 (patient with insomnia). In the third extract, a nurse manager commented on the perceived existence of the problem when discussing Vignette 3 (parents who complained) a vignette in which the assessment phase was deliberately omitted):

'The patient denies she has any other problems so the sister leaves it at that. She doesn't investigate further than that'.

'I would have tried to find out if there are any other reasons why she is not sleeping other than what it says here, personal worries, family worries, financial problems . . .'

'I'm not sure that the tactics were right. It implies, because the sister apologised to the parents, it implies poor nursing care. There may well have been a problem, but the facts haven't been established.'

15. The most appropriate assessor

A few informants (8), three of whom were nurse managers, commented on the person they felt was the most appropriate assessor. In most cases, it was suggested that the nurse who had been assigned to a patient would be the natural person to assess that patient. This point is highlighted in the quotation below, which came from a nurse teacher discussing Vignette 4 (patient who has undergone enucleation):

> 'My immediate reaction to this was to ask if the sister was the right person to be assessing him after being away for two weeks. With this patient being almost ready for discharge I thought perhaps she was the wrong person. There is no mention of the nurse who has already been involved with the patient.'

What made a nurse the appropriate assessor was first-hand knowledge of and rapport with the patient.

It was felt that the patient should set the agenda for the assessment with the nurse. All who mentioned this believed that such collaboration would improve the quality of the data.

16. Assessment skills

Generally, these skills were said to be related to clinical experience, a point made especially by the more experienced informants. Occasionally, specific assessment skills were mentioned; for example, a nurse teacher highlighted negotiating skills when discussing Vignette 7 (patient with diabetes):

> 'The assessment has been good in this. There has been mutual negotiation. The sister has also listened carefully to the patient as to what the actual problem is, and that is a strength as such.'

17. Two-stage and multi-stage assessment

There were instances when informants (particularly quite a high proportion (58 per cent) of nurse managers) felt that a single assessment would have been inappropriate. Some favoured an early, rapid assessment to identify the problem(s), followed by a deeper assessment to provide a more detailed picture. For example, a nurse manager (discussing Vignette 1, patient with insomnia) said:

> 'The first assessment should have identified those factors included at the second assessment. The second assessment should have been used to find out more about her problems. The sister is not skilled as an assessor.'

Others, however, described another type of assessment, what might be called an *ad hoc* assessment, necessary when a nurse is faced with an unexpected problem. Even then it was suggested that the underlying problem should be quickly identified, followed by a more detailed assessment. That is, assessment becomes a two-stage process.

In other cases, some informants felt it appropriate to carry out a second or third assessment at the end of a problem-solving sequence. A few considered evaluation and assessment together; that is, once the effects of the nursing interventions had been evaluated, another assessment should be undertaken to identify further problems. Others, however, disagreed with this strategy, explaining that all the patient's problems should be listed as actual or potential problems at the initial assessment.

Summary of the assessment phase

The views and statements on assessment in this study support the literature as follows:

1. assessment is an important activity in clinical problem-solving. It is the phase in which patient-related data are collected and analysed (Johnson et al., 1980, pp. 56–7);
2. nurses use their experiences to help them draw conclusions from assessment information (Johnson et al., 1980, p. 72); and there appears to be a relationship between the level of experience and the form of the interpretation;
3. weak assessments are characterised by poor data collection and data classification (Aspinall, 1976; Corcoran, 1986);
4. assessment enables the nurse to understand the problem in relation to the patient and his or her other problems (Vitale et al., 1978, pp. 38–46);
5. nurses appear to spend some time interpreting assessment data before deciding what other information is required, and data can come from a variety of sources (Johnson et al., 1980, p. 72);
6. assessment may involve the patient by seeking his or her views on the problem. Other health-care workers can also contribute to a nursing assessment (Lauri, 1982);
7. assessment data may need to be corroborated in certain circumstances (Johnson et al., 1980, p. 72);
8. timing of the assessment is important to the problem-solving process (Bailey and Claus, 1975, p. 21);
9. assessment seems to be at least a two-staged process which may consist of a general assessment to identify problems, followed by an in-depth problem-specific assessment (Bailey and Claus, 1975, p. 22; Johnson et al., 1980, 56–7; Barker, 1987).

No significant new insights emerged from this analysis of views and statements on assessment.

3. Planning

Much less discussion took place on planning than with assessment and implementation. This is surprising in view of the emphasis and importance attached to planning in recent literature (see Johnson et al., 1980, pp. 75–95; Barnett, 1985; Buckenham, 1986; Filkins, 1986; Hardy and Engel, 1987). When discussion took place it was detailed and some strong views were expressed. From an analysis of interview transcripts, responses fell into nine categories.

18. Relationship between planning and assessment

Informants reflected on assessment statements to help them judge the relevance and quality of the plan. The two quotations that follow show the relationship between planning and assessment. The first was a comment from a staff nurse discussing Vignette 1 (patient with insomnia) and the second from a sister discussing Vignette 6 (patient with a circulatory problem):

> 'She went to the patient and tried to discover what was wrong and to get to the root of the problem. She then designed her care plan around that assessment.'

> 'The patient has said that his arm is painful. I didn't think she assessed him too well. She didn't look exactly where the pain was coming from; whether it was the wound site, or whether it was the plaster compressing his arm. So, rather than making a more refined assessment she immediately went straight in and cut the Velband, rather than planning her actions more carefully upon what the cause could be and what she could do about that particular cause. So, I felt that her plan wasn't brilliant and her assessment was less than useless.'

The relationship between planning and assessment was particularly clear in the discussion of Vignette 2 where the sister had developed a nursing plan to assist wound healing without first assessing the patient, or indeed, seeing the wound. This is illustrated in the comment below from a staff nurse:

> 'It seems that the sister sets the goals for this particular patient's care without actually going to see him and finding out what his problems are. As soon as she is told of a problem she writes down the goals before she actually does something. You would go and take a wound swab at least.'

Surprisingly, there was a lack of discussion about standard care plans which, according to information from several nurses, feature in the wards in most of the Districts from which the majority of the informants were drawn. Standard care plans are an efficient way of documenting the care a patient will need, and consist of the nursing interventions which are commonly required for the majority of patients on a particular ward; for example, the accepted pre-operative and post-operative care on a surgical ward. One reason why informants failed to discuss this may have been because the focus of the interviews was clinical problem-solving and not the nursing process, which is more usually associated with standard care plans.

19. Summarising the plan

As in the case of problem identification and assessment, some informants spent time summarising the description of the plan in the vignettes. Their discussion of planning tended to fall into two parts: (1) the goals; and (2) the nursing interventions to achieve the goals. Sometimes they even did this when discussing Vignettes 3 and 7, which did not include planning. In the first quotation below a nurse manager discussed only the goals when referring to Vignette 5 (patient with angina), and in the second a nurse teacher considered both the goals and interventions when referring to Vignette 1 (patient with insomnia):

> 'The goals are good but are lacking in detail. The health education goal is good though.'

> 'The interventions in the care plan were very nice and relate to the goals, especially the one about the patient's bed being placed in the side room to ensure quietness. I thought that was very good and considerate of the sister.'

As we shall see, discussion of the 'goal' and the 'nursing intervention' components of planning becomes a recurrent theme throughout this section.

20. Quality judgements in planning

As in the case of assessment (Category 9 (p. 80) quality judgements in assessment), some informants judged the quality of the plan. This is evident in the following two quotations. The first came from a sister discussing Vignette 5 (patient with angina), and the second from a nurse manager discussing Vignette 4 (patient who has undergone enucleation):

> 'I think this is a good care plan because the goals are good.'

'I thought it was a considerate, compassionate and well thought-out care plan in that it looked at clinical nursing problems as well as psychological problems.'

Planning was also felt to be good when written plans (a) were based on the assessment of the patient; (b) included clear goals and interventions; (c) were logically set out; and (d) included the patient and family in the planning process.

Planning was criticised when written plans (a) missed out problems or goals or interventions; (b) were out of date; (c) included goals that could not be measured; and (d) had not been prepared by the nurse who assessed the patient.

21. The problem component

The plan was occasionally discussed in relation to the patient's problems particularly when the identification of the problem was criticised. An example of this category can be seen below in the quotation from a sister discussing Vignette 3 (parents who complained):

'The care plan and actions are inappropriate since the true problems have not been identified.'

22. The goal component

This was the most frequently discussed issue in planning, attracting comment uniformly from about 75 per cent of each of the groups of practitioners. Goals were specifically mentioned in five of the seven vignettes, and when goals were incorporated informants spoke at length about them. For example, a charge nurse focused on the goals in Vignette 6 (patient with a circulatory problem):

'I like the fact that the sister set three important short-term goals for this patient. Clearly, it would seem like a situation which I would think reasonably and regularly occurs in orthopaedic-surgical wards, where post-operative complications of this kind occur in vascular surgery. They do occur, although it isn't being handled like a crisis at the time, but certainly it is an important problem. The patient is going to be anxious about it. It is going to develop serious complications if nothing is done about it and something isn't done immediately about it. So I think she has highlighted three important goals to overcome a serious problem.'

In general, goals that were perceived as clear, realistic, achievable and had the patient's agreement were praised. Those felt too separated from a nursing intervention or seen as unmeasurable were criticised.

Some informants commented on the prioritising of goals and this seemed to depend on many factors; for example, in the case of Vignette 4 (patient who has undergone enucleation), it was felt that psychological goals ought to take priority over the clinical ones as in the case of the sister who commented on Vignette 4:

'The goals are set down wrongly. The psychological goals are the priority
. . .'

Goals were categorised in other ways too, the commonest was to label them as short- or long-term. Other forms of classification were (a) attachment of goals to previously identified problems; and (b) establishing the main goal and sub-goals. The following quotation illustrates concern for long- and short-term goals and came from a charge nurse discussing Vignette 1 (patient with insomnia):

'Once again, the discussion which took place with the doctor led to the setting of two goals which are not stated to be either long- or short-term.'

23.   The intervention component

With the exception of staff nurses, some members of all groups of informants contended that the relationship between interventions and goals was unclear and some vignettes did not indicate how goals would be achieved, as seen in the following comments. The first two came from a charge nurse and nurse teacher respectively, discussing Vignette 5 (patient with angina), and the third from a sister discussing Vignette 2 (patient with an inflamed wound):

'The plan seems ideal. It is essential that the patient loses weight and stops smoking, etc. But it doesn't clearly indicate how this will be achieved . . .'

'The nurses seem to have got the plan confused. Very often they do not say how the goals will be achieved, for example, "this patient should reduce her smoking by ten cigarettes a week and do this by recording her daily total". Goals and means of achieving them should be distinguishable.'

'She hasn't actually said how she will go about doing that. It is just a goal stuck on its own. There is no mention of the care plan being changed. It is usual to write an intervention alongside a goal.'

24.   Role of patient and others

The role of the patient in planning interventions attracted comment from more than half of the informants, particularly a high proportion of nurse teachers (71 per cent). The inclusion of the patient in this process was seen as positive and exclusion was criticised. Examples are given below, the first extract came from a sister discussing Vignette 5 (patient with angina) and the second from a nurse teacher discussing Vignette 7 (patient with diabetes):

'The plan has been set with the patient's agreement and that is fine. You can't just blunder through saying she's got to diet, she's got to stop smoking. You have got to have a chat with her on how she feels about her condition, prognosis, family history, and does it bother her. Does she feel she wants to do something about it. You have, first of all, got to get an agreement, a positive attitude from the patient otherwise you have no right to impose and decide for her. It is still her decision isn't it if she is going to make any effort to improve things.'

'I am reiterating again, but she has not negotiated with the patient . . . in terms of what the care is going to be. She has moved directly into implementation of the care.'

Informants went on to suggest that the plans which had involved the patient were more precise, more realistic and more likely to be successful than where the patient was excluded. Some explained that if the patient had brought the problem to the sister's attention, then it was logical to allow the patient to suggest or agree on the plan of action. Much discussion centred on the way the patient could help in goal-setting and some felt that the patient and the nurse should jointly determine what independent contribution the patient could make.

Some informants thought it logical that other staff with specialist knowledge would contribute to the plan. These included the infection control sister, doctor, dietician, health visitor, district nurse, physiotherapist, occupational therapist and social worker. Some, however, felt that other health professionals should be 'watched' in case they 'take over' or 'usurp the ward nurse's responsibility'! In short, while informants welcomed specialist advice, some were protective of the ward nurse's perceived role. The following extracts from interviews with learner nurses (discussing Vignette 5, patient with angina) show first, a positive view, and second, a more cautious view towards multidisciplinary planning:

'When the sister is planning the care the patient is to receive, I like the way she involves all members of the team, the physician, dietician, and other nurses as well.'

'Although the nurse and the physician work along side, I do think at the end of the day it should be the nurses who plan and carry out her nursing care. I am not anti-doctor, but it is the nurses who are with the patient far more than any other person, and they are going to get to know the patient a lot more. The patient would be able to talk to them and get a good rapport with them.'

25. Nursing experience in planning

A small number of informants commented on the importance of the length and type of nursing experience in planning. For example, a sister, commented on the type of experience in Vignette 2 (patient with an inflamed wound), by saying:

'Because the problem wasn't assessed or confirmed, the care given seems unnecessary. Sister is relying on clinical experience when planning the care.'

Informants also stated that the job of deciding priorities in the plan was a skilled one that comes with experience, and that correctly ordered goals would help a less experienced nurse to deliver a patient's care. However, a few informants pointed out the educational value of involving learner nurses in the planning process. As one staff nurse commented when discussing Vignette 2 (patient with an inflamed wound):

'Once again, the problem has been tackled well, but I thought that the student nurse should have set the goals which the sister could have gone over with her.'

26.   Place of medical treatment

Some informants (commonly sisters) felt that the plan in certain vignettes was based on a medical model in that investigation, diagnosis, and treatment had influenced the plan. In the quotation below, a charge nurse, discussing Vignette 1 (patient with insomnia), was critical of a plan felt to have been influenced by a medical model:

'The care plan seems very medically-oriented, "The surgeon orders the wound swab". A great deal of it seems to be about medical problems, very unclear without specific nursing instruction.'

Medical treatment was not seen to be an important part of the nursing plan by any informant. However, one recently qualified staff nurse noted that the plan had not been sanctioned by a doctor and was, therefore, inappropriate. In discussing Vignette 6 (patient with a circulatory problem), she said:

'The nurse decides on what is to be done although the doctor hasn't been asked, or even decided what the problem is. Not knowing what the problem is, how can you decide on what care needs to be given? It is the doctor's decision on what needs to be done not the nurse's.'

The informant's limited and specific experience in an intensive care unit may be a factor influencing her fairly strong views.

Summary of the planning phase

The number of comments on planning (333) were greater than those relating to problem identification and evaluation, but were easily outnumbered by problem assessment and implementation. It is difficult to explain this, but possibly nurses place more emphasis on assessing and implementing than planning. Further research is needed to confirm and clarify this point. The views and statements on planning in this study support the literature as follows:

1. the planning phase is logically related to the assessment which precedes it. The problem or problems arising from the assessment do appear to be a focus for planning (Johnson et al., 1980, p. 144; McCarthy, 1981);
2. the goals and interventions making up the plan are prioritised in some way (Vitale et al., 1978, p. 8);
3. the plan consists of two components; the goal to be achieved and the intervention required to reach the goal (Kron, 1966, p. 141; Bailey and Claus, 1975, pp. 25–6);
4. the patient and other health-care workers have an important role in the planning phase (Vitale et al., 1978, pp. 8–9);
5. planning relies to some extent on the nurse's experience (Barnett, 1985);
6. there is a relationship between the planning process and nursing autonomy (Hammond, 1966).

The literature is less well supported in the following ways:

1. the sample of practitioners in this research, when reviewing the given plans, did not appear to identify alternative interventions in addition to their preferred interventions as mentioned by Bailey and Claus (1975, pp. 25–6);
2. medical treatments were generally not recognised by practitioners as part of the nursing plan. Although the medical model, as a basis for planning, is supported by Johnson et al. (1980, p. 78), it is eschewed by most nurses in this study.

As we saw in Chapter 6 and again in this chapter, the construction of a plan has not attracted as much attention from the informants as some writers think it deserves.

4. Implementation

There were more comments (593) on implementation than any other phase. Indeed, views and statements on implementation well outnumbered its nearest rival (problem assessment). Twelve categories of response emerge from an analysis of the informants' extensive discussion.

27. Summarising implementation

As we have seen in preceding phases, an early activity for many informants was to summarise the stated implementation phase. This can be seen in the following extract which came from an interview with a nurse teacher discussing Vignette 7 (patient with diabetes):

> 'Initially, she reassures him, which is a quite normal action. She doesn't sound too patronising. She also involves the family which I think is one of the most important things. I think she must have explained all about it to them too. Also the ex-patient – getting him to talk. The dietician determines the patient's nutritional requirements . . .'

28. Judging the quality of implementation

In reflecting on the vignettes, many informants (including all the learner nurses) agreed or disagreed with the nurses' actions, and this category attracted the most comment. Their discussion tended to consist of simple statements; for example, a sister who commented positively on Vignette 4 (patient who has undergone enucleation) said:

> 'I liked the way they place great emphasis on getting him to accept his prosthesis.'

There were slightly more informants (again, a high proportion of learner nurses) who disagreed with the stated interventions, and these comments tended to be longer. For example, in contrast to the length and type of comment in the quotation above, a learner nurse criticising the care in Vignette 4 said:

> 'The sister is more interested in the skin around the socket and how he is going to look after it has healed and after the prosthesis is in. I thought that was a bit too clinical and not enough emphasis placed on psychological care.'

Other examples of quality judgements can be seen in Category 27 (summarising implementation) and Category 30 (timing and sequencing of interventions).

29. Alternative and/or additional interventions

Some informants recommended alternative interventions when commenting on the implementation phase. The additional suggested interventions took various forms. For example, one type of comment was on alternative action, that is, some informants preferred to substitute the stated intervention with another. Others felt that an additional strategy was required in case the main one failed. At other times it was suggested that a goal might be better achieved by alternating between intervention strategies. In this extract a sister, in discussing Vignette 2 (patient with an inflamed wound), suggested an alternative intervention thus:

'I would have found some other way of feeding him. It doesn't say he had an intravenous infusion, or how he was getting fluids. I certainly would have looked into that . . .'

30.   Timing and sequencing of interventions

Comments on the optimal timing of nursing interventions were common. In the first of the two extracts below, a learner nurse commented on Vignette 1 (patient with insomnia) and in the second, a staff nurse discussed Vignette 4 (patient who has undergone enucleation):

'I felt there ought to have been more counselling at night when it would have been more effective; also the nurse would have had more time at night. What they did wasn't wrong, but you have got to organise these things better. I do think that could have been done at night.'

'He may never accept his injury ever. I think he is very bitter about what has happened. At that point [points to top of list], someone should have been brought in, someone with a similar injury and not left till the end. If that patient [with a similar problem] is brought in very early, then he may accept it a little better, but to see another patient, just before he goes home is very bad management.'

Another group of comments was on the 'running order', that is, the sequence in which the nursing interventions should be implemented. An interesting feature was the diversity of ways in which informants ordered the nursing interventions. One was to implement them in relation to the way goals in the plan were prioritised. Another way was to order them independently of the plan where experience seemed to be a guiding influence. The following quotations demonstrate these points. Both came from nurses discussing Vignette 2 (patient with an inflamed wound). The first came from a nurse teacher and the second from a staff nurse.

'His mouth care should be earlier in the list, because it would not only improve his comfort and minimise infection, it would also improve his appetite. Therefore, he could take a high protein diet to improve wound healing.'

'I would have the patient's level of discomfort first on the list, then his vital signs. Then you would have the explanations to Mr Franks and his wife nearer the bottom. I feel that it is very important to put his temperature near the top, and I certainly would have dealing with the relatives near the bottom.'

The first quotation is without doubt goal-related, while the second appears to be experience-related.

In urgent situations it was suggested that the whole problem-solving process should be re-ordered to overcome a problem. For example, in the case of the circulatory problem in Vignette 6, the existing strategy of problem identification, assessment, planning and implementation would be inappropriate. Rather, the nurse should implement a solution based on a quick assessment, followed by the construction of a detailed plan after a more in-depth investigation. In other words, the problem-solving sequence would be: (1) problem identification; (2) rapid assessment; (3) implementation of solution; (4) detailed assessment; (5) planning; (6) implementation of further actions; and (7) evaluation (to be discussed later).

Other examples of the suggested change in the sequence of problem-solving are highlighted in the quotations below. The first came from a sister discussing Vignette 3 (parents who complained), the second from a nurse teacher discussing Vignette 4 (patient who has undergone enucleation), and the third from a learner nurse discussing Vignette 7 (patient with diabetes):

'I would have asked the parents to come to a quiet room, then calm them down. I would ensure that the nappy is being changed, then I would investigate the problem and identify any other problems. I would investigate the nappy problem to see if there was a problem at all.'

'The specific care is OK. However, the ex-patient should have been brought in much earlier to give him more encouragement. The self-care part also brought in earlier, as soon as the shock of the injury is over. It could be part of the assessment really.'

'I don't think we started teaching quick enough. It should have been go from the time when he came in really. Unless he was too ill of course.'

31. Role of patient, relative and ex-patient

As we saw in problem identification (Category 6, confirming the problem), in problem assessment (Categories 12 and 13, confirming assessment data and timing of assessment respectively) and in planning (Category 24, role of patient and others) the role of the patient in implementation was frequently discussed. More than half of the informants, and in particular a high proportion of learner nurses (73 per cent), commented on the part the patient and, additionally in some cases, a relative or relatives could play.

The extensive discussion can be summarised into three parts. First, some informants suggested that patients could be given responsibility for part or even all the care. For example, a nurse manager discussing Vignette 7 (patient with diabetes) commented:

'Sometimes we impose our care on patients too much. We should give back to him some responsibility for his own care. The nurse has tried to do this to a certain extent, but not enough.'

Most of these suggestions were, however, qualified with a statement that the nurse should supervise the patient at all times. Second, it was felt that relatives have a role to play in implementation, particularly when the patient required continuation of care at home. Third, it was suggested that ex-patients could contribute to care by bringing special knowledge and skills to help the patient overcome a problem.

32. Role of other health workers

The place of medical decisions in the planning phase was discussed earlier (see Category 24, role of patient and others). In the implementation phase, the role of the doctor was also discussed. Informants felt that some nursing interventions either led to medical intervention, or came about directly as a consequence of the medical investigation and treatment. For example, the quotation below, from a sister commenting on Vignette 7 (patient with diabetes), highlighted the close relationship between medical treatment and nursing care when nurses were making slow progress with the rehabilitation of a patient who is unable to administer his insulin:

'She must tell the physician of the patient's difficulties because he needs to know. He may well say "let's leave it [the education programme] for the moment, let him [the patient] do what he can, then we will adjust his insulin to get a better balance".'

Informants were divided approximately equally as to whether doctors should have to agree to certain nursing actions. One group felt that the nurse should not implement the plan until the doctor's permission had been obtained. As we saw in Category 26 (place of medical treatments), these were the less experienced nurses who were talking about the more medically-oriented situations such as the circulatory problem in Vignette 6. On the other hand, as in the case of Category 24 (role of patient and others), some informants held strong views about the nurse's autonomy in planning, and this held for implementing solutions to nursing problems as well. Another group, however, perceived the necessity for nurses to inform the doctor of the nursing strategy, because of the doctor's responsibility for the patient. Some informants obviously enjoyed a good working relationship with their medical colleagues and welcomed medical views on nursing actions. It was generally agreed that medical and nursing care could not be separated, because any medical instruction having a bearing on the problem or goal ought to be implemented along with the nursing care.

It was also felt that other health professionals may have a role in implementation. Such people would bring special skills to overcome the problem; for example, a sister commenting on Vignette 7 (patient with diabetes) explained:

> 'By using the dietician and the diabetic liaison people, he is going to get better answers if he has more in-depth questions. They are obviously going to handle the answers better.'

33. Role of planning/goals

There were regular attempts to trace nursing interventions back to the plan, especially by sisters. For example, one sister, when discussing Vignette 4 (patient who has undergone enucleation), said:

> 'The interventions do not match the priorities set in terms of the goals. The nursing care would have been much clearer if the actions had been grouped according to the goals.'

But informants' discussion of the implementation phase was sometimes unrelated to the goals in the nursing plan, and it appeared that such comments were made from experience; that is, they were based on the informant's encounters with similar problems, recalled through the stimulus of the vignette. This was particularly true when informants disagreed with the given interventions. For example, the following quotation came from a charge nurse discussing Vignette 3 (parents who complained):

> 'I think the sister was wrong to immediately apologise and say that the occurrence will not happen again. What I would have suggested was apologise and say that this could have happened any time . . . So I would have thought the sister should have gone to the parents and reassured them about that.'

34. Role of the problem

Interventions were sometimes discussed directly in relation to the problem taking no account of the plan. For example, in the first extract below, a sister discussed Vignette 4 (patient who has undergone enucleation). In the second a learner nurse commented on Vignette 6 (patient with a circulatory problem) and in the third a charge nurse reflected upon Vignette 1 (patient with insomnia):

> 'Specific care has been given to areas identified as worrying John, that is, appearance, support at home and follow-up care.'

'Because his fingers were swollen, blue, cold and painful, an important thing would have been to elevate the arm.'

'I think that placing the patient in the sideroom . . . would be one way of dealing with the problem.'

35. Role of assessment

There were also occasions when interventions were discussed in relation to assessment data, again without reference to the plan. The following extracts highlight this issue. The first quotation came from a sister discussing Vignette 7 (patient with diabetes) and the second came from a sister discussing Vignette 5 (patient with angina). The third came from a charge nurse commenting on Vignette 3 (parents who complained):

'She has done a very thorough assessment there. She knows what to do and she takes immediate action by reassuring him . . .'

'She is still working at the age of 59. She is married with a family. Could she take early retirement? Could she get redundancy pay? That sort of thing.'

'I'm a little concerned that the sister apologises to the parents as if what they are saying is correct. There may be other reasons behind their complaint about the baby's care.'

36. Role of ward routine

A few informants (sisters and learner nurses only) criticised the nursing actions in the vignettes which were said to be 'ward routine' or 'ritualistic', rather than being tailored to the patient's needs. For example, in the extracts below, a sister and learner nurse respectively, criticised the care given in Vignette 2 (patient with an inflamed wound):

'I couldn't see the point of doing mouth care . . . That shouldn't have been a specific thing. That should have been something of a norm anyway . . . routine to the problem.'

'I thought it [the care] was too ritualistic. Getting his antibiotic changed, having one team looking after him, his diet and all that. It is set out ritualistically, not at all individualised . . .'

In reflecting on this category and the previous three categories, it is not altogether clear why informants used a goal or a problem to explain an intervention, but it does seem to be related to experience. From this research it appears that some interventions based solely on an analysis of the problem, or an assessment, or on routine procedures do not particularly need a written plan.

37. Educational value of implementation for learners

A little over one third of the informants (35 per cent) commented on the educational value of the implementation phase for learner nurses. Views and statements often centred on opportunities for the learner nurse to participate. For example, a manager when discussing Vignette 3 (parents who complained), said:

> 'She [the sister] should have supported the learner in this situation rather than taking over from her in dealing with the parents . . .'

Informants also commented on the educational value of the other problem-solving phases (particularly planning, see Category 25, nursing experience in planning) but not to the extent of the discussion here.

38. Recording nursing interventions

The importance of written and verbal communication was mentioned by some informants when commenting on the implementation phase. For example, a learner nurse discussing Vignette 3 (parents who complained) explained:

> 'I was impressed with the communications on the ward. The sister is keen on recording things. She makes a formal report and she passes it on to the next shift. Because she has explained, they are all in the picture.'

Accurate recordings were felt to be particularly important in cases of untoward incidents.

Summary of the implementation phase

The views and statements on implementation in this study support the literature in the following ways:

1. implementing the plan is an important part of clinical problem solving (Johnson et al., 1980, pp. 87–8). Informants made more comments on implementation than on any other phase;
2. prioritising and timing of interventions is an important part of problem-solving (Vitale et al., 1978, pp. 83–7). Specific interventions may need to be implemented even before a thorough assessment has been done, particularly in urgent situations (Johnson et al., 1980, p. 7);
3. implementing the plan can involve the patient, relative(s), and other health workers (Vitale et al., 1978, pp. 83–7);
4. medical treatment having a bearing on nursing interventions are implemented in parallel with the nursing interventions (Johnson et al., 1980, pp. 80–4);

5. nurses draw on their knowledge and experience when considering how and when nursing interventions are implemented (Johnson et al., 1980, p. 87). Nurses may use experience to solve a problem and not refer to the plan (Miller, 1984);
6. the implementation phase is felt to have educational value for learner nurses (Priestley et al., 1979, p. 70);
7. accurate recording of nursing interventions is an important process in the implementation phase (Kron, 1966, p. 65).

This research indicates that nursing interventions are not always goal-based and this finding, therefore, is not in accordance with the views of Johnson et al. (1980, pp. 87–8). Rather, it would seem that in some cases interventions may be problem-based, routine-based, experience-based or largely intuitive.

5. Evaluation

Evaluation, surprisingly, attracted less attention than assessment, planning and implementation. From an analysis of the transcripts, thirteen categories of response emerge.

39. Summarising evaluation

The informant's habit of summarising the phase under discussion also occurred in evaluation. Almost a third of the informants (30 per cent) paraphrased the written account to help them focus on evaluation. In the first extract a staff nurse commented on Vignette 3 (parents who complained), and in the second a sister discussed Vignette 5 (patient with angina):

'Certainly, things seem to get better as they are sorted out. The parents are much happier, they greet the nurse a lot more friendlier . . .'

'The patient is confident she is going to stop smoking. She realises the need to eat a healthier diet. The family are going to support. There isn't much more you can do.'

40. Quality judgements in evaluation

Generally, informants' comments on the quality of the evauation process were single bold value statements such as 'the evaluation is good' or 'the evaluation is poor'. Occasionally, the informant would give a rationale for his or her judgement of the evaluation phase and this is implicit within some of the quotations discussed later; for example, see Category 42 (evaluation issues) and Category 46 (a means of determining patient's progress).

41. Assessment as a synonym for evaluation

Interestingly, within the process of summarising, seven informants used 'assessment' as a synonym for evaluation. At least one member from each group, with the exception of nurse teachers, did this. In the first quotation, a nurse manager made the statement when discussing Vignette 5 (patient with angina). In the second example a sister, discussing Vignette 6 (patient with a circulatory problem), made a similar statement:

> 'The goals were good. The first was to reduce her anxiety. Having said that, there is no evidence that they assessed to actually see if they achieved that goal.'

> 'They make his arm comfortable. It is put in a comfortable position and then they deal with the pain. Then they assess the effect of the analgesia they have decided to give. She should re-assess at a time when she thinks the analgesic should have been effective. If it hasn't, then she should ask the doctor to change the medication to something more effective . . .'

Although the terms are used interchangeably by lay persons, in professional contexts, such as nursing and education, they have different meanings. If the terms are used synonymously in nursing, in any verbal or written communication, there may be confusion.

42. Evaluation issues

Many informants (65) from all groups focused on particular evaluation issues when deciding if the whole or part of the problem had been solved. Comments within this category were far more numerous than in any other evaluation category and may be sub-categorised into four areas:

1. evaluation of the nursing plan;
2. evaluation of goals;
3. evaluation of the patient's problem;
4. other specific issues in evaluation.

The following selection of extracts from interviews illustrate informants' concerns.
   1. Evaluation of the nursing plan
   This was highlighted by a learner nurse who discussed Vignette 1 (patient with insomnia):

'You would do a care plan each day and evaluate it every one or two days, rather than twice a day. Obviously, if there was something really important, then I would evaluate the care plan every day.'

2. Evaluation of goals

This was indicated by a sister who commented on Vignette 7 (patient with diabetes):

'The reason the evaluation is not detailed enough is that the sister didn't set any goals in the first place. She hasn't got any goals to evaluate.'

3. Evaluation of the patient's problem

A charge nurse discussing Vignette 4 (patient who has undergone enucleation) said:

'Of all the vignettes I have discussed so far, this is the only one where I feel that the problem hasn't been evaluated. I feel that the patient may have gone home with a problem still existing.'

4. Other specific issues in evaluation

An example of such an issue would be measuring the patient's temperature as a means of determining his or her progress. Other examples of specific concerns can be seen in a comment from a nurse teacher also discussing Vignette 4:

'When he goes home, it just says that he goes home. It doesn't say that he was fully evaluated. Evaluation of the care he has had, whether the staff feel happy about him going home. How does he feel about going home? How will he cope with his socket and prosthesis? How does he feel about going back to work? These are some of the things I would check.'

Some informants evaluated in a very broad sense by judging the overall outcome in relation to the plan only. Others were more specific in that they examined the effects of interventions on the goal or on the patient's problem. The choice of approach, as we have seen with other aspects of problem-solving, appears to be based on experience and dependent on the context of the problem.

43. Frequency of evaluation

There appeared to be a relationship between the type of problem (or goal) and the frequency of evaluation. In the case of a problem, it was felt (perhaps predictably) that urgent ones, such as the circulatory problem, require continuous monitoring, while long-term ones need only a weekly evaluation. When evaluation focused on the goal a similar relationship emerged. For example, it was suggested that a sleep goal should be evaluated daily, whereas a target-weight goal should be evaluated weekly.

In short, it would seem that the frequency of evaluation is related to the rate of physiological and/or psychological change associated with the patient's problem or goal. An example of a learner nurse commenting on the frequency of evaluation occurred in Vignette 5 (patient with angina):

> 'It says that ten days later she [the sister] checks the records. It indicates to me that she hasn't been taking much notice of her [the patient]. She hasn't been checking on a day-to-day basis what weight she has lost and what success she has with cutting down her cigarettes . . .'

44. Role of nurse and other health workers

As in the case of assessment in Category 15 (the most appropriate assessor), the nurse most closely associated with the patient's problem (for example, the primary nurse) was felt to be the most appropriate evaluator. The statement below came from a staff nurse discussing Vignette 2 (patient with an inflamed wound) who advocated evaluation by the primary nurse:

> 'His vital signs were recorded four hourly, body temperature and that sort of thing. The wound is re-dressed daily by the same nurse so that we get a truer picture. If you have got different nurses doing it, you don't always see whether there is an improvement.'

Informants also said that there should be associate evaluators whose role might be to confirm the main evaluator's findings. Such associate evaluators could be a nurse on the opposite shift, a medical or paramedical colleague.

It was also suggested that the patient's progress could be evaluated at a multidisciplinary team meeting (sometimes referred to as a case conference). The solving of clinical problems tends to involve more than one discipline and case conferences would examine the issue in an efficient manner. For these informants evaluation is not solely the nurse's responsibility.

45. Role of patient, parent and family

It was sometimes stated that the patient and relatives may also have a role in the evaluation phase; that is, they might be asked directly for views on progress. The quotations below highlight this concern. In the first extract, a nurse teacher, discussing Vignette 1 (patient with insomnia), considered the patient's involvement, and in the second quotation a sister discussing Vignette 4 (patient who has undergone enucleation) focused on the parent:

> 'I mean, to end it by saying that the patient's stay is uneventful . . . that doesn't follow the pattern at all. That may be how the nurses perceive it. I would suggest that the patient wouldn't perceive it that way.'

'The sister doesn't go back and talk to the mother. It was the mother who pointed out the problem. She doesn't use the mother as an evaluator, which might help.'

46.   A means of determining patient's progress

It appears that evaluation serves several functions within a five-phase model of problem-solving. However, some members of each group of informants (with the exception of managers) remarked that an important function was to help the nurse decide on the progress made as well as on whether the problem had been solved. This is formative and summative evaluation although these terms were not used by the informants.

Two examples of judging progress follow. The first came from a nurse teacher discussing Vignette 6 (patient with a circulatory problem), and the second came from a learner nurse discussing Vignette 3 (parents who complained):

'I would have cut the Velband to make sure the swelling reduced. If it didn't then I would get the nurse to check him every fifteen minutes in the hour. It doesn't say she has done that. So that is the only thing I would criticise this one for.'

'Then she follows it up again constantly . . . ensuring, keeping an eye on the parents. Making sure that things are running smoothly, and problems are not cropping up. There is an element of evaluation here.'

47.   A means of judging the plan or action

This category attracted a lot of comment, including the majority of learner nurses (59 per cent). Some informants stated that evaluation should be used to judge the appropriateness of the care plan previously set and pointed out that the care plan may need to be updated following evalua-tion. Updating may include modification of nursing interventions designed to achieve elements of the care plan. The following quotation highlights these issues and came from a teacher discussing Vignette 1 (patient with insomnia):

'Changes are made to the patient's care plan and then implemented – not just paying lip-service to it. Another evaluation is made of the new care plan . . .'

Informants from all groups commented on another function of evaluation – judging the success of an intervention. One of the informants (a staff nurse), who commented in this way when discussing Vignette 1 (patient with insomnia), said:

'As a result of her [the sister's] actions, the problem appears to have been solved and no further action seems necessary.'

Interestingly, some informants also used evaluation to suggest new interventions without particular reference to planning. For example, when commenting on Vignette 5 (patient with angina), a sister said:

'Since the patient has only reduced her smoking and not stopped, I feel the nursing care has not been positive enough. There hasn't been enough counselling by staff.'

This is perhaps not surprising since, as we saw earlier, informants sometimes discussed implementation without reference to a plan.

48.   A means of identifying new problems

Another function of evaluation was the detection of new problems. The link between evaluation and problem identification was discussed by twelve informants, who identified fresh problems when discussing evaluation. One of the twelve (a charge nurse), when discussing Vignette 1, (patient with insomnia) explained:

'Her care has been evaluated well, and the sister further tries to help by identifying any other problems which seem not to be apparent.'

49.   Assessment following evaluation

A small number of informants (10) demonstrated a cyclical approach to their problem-solving by returning to the assessment following evaluation. In the quotations below, a learner nurse, commenting on Vignette 5 (patient with angina), and a sister, discussing Vignette 3 (parents who complained), illustrated the need for further investigation following evaluation:

'The only thing was the smoking. They couldn't reduce her smoking. She couldn't do what she was asked. I thought that could have been investigated a bit more.'

'What's on paper obviously worked, and she checked that the parents were reassured. If I was the sister here, I would want to investigate what actually happened over the past eight hours . . .'

50.   Evaluation in the sequence of problem-solving

Six informants placed evaluation within a named sequence of problem-solving, usually when concluding their discussion of a vignette. For example, a nurse teacher when commenting on Vignette 6 (patient with a circulatory problem) outlined a linear, step-wise phase model of problem solving ending with evaluation:

> 'The action she has taken actually followed a logical path. She looked at his arm, assessed there was a problem. She has done something about that problem, with the plan she has given. She obviously has implemented some care and then evaluated it.'

51. Recording and communicating evaluation evidence

A smaller number of informants (9) commented on recording and communicating the evaluation process than was the case with the implementation phase (Category 38, recording nursing interventions, N = 35). The quotation below came from a staff nurse discussing Vignette 2 (patient with an inflamed wound):

> 'At the bottom it says daily written and verbal reports are made. I'm not sure that is necessary. They should be setting the evaluation of a goal for a week's time, for example, 'the wound will be X much better', rather than writing daily reports. You wouldn't really gain much from doing it daily.'

Comment was made about the importance of accurate recording of information in the case of an untoward incident, and the educational and practical benefits of full and clear reporting to colleagues.

Summary of the evaluation phase

The views and statements on evaluation in this study support the literature in the following ways:

1. assessment and evaluation are used synonymously by some nurses when describing evaluation (Vitale et al., 1978, p. 85; Roper et al., 1983, p. 14);
2. the evaluation criterion may be as broad as the plan, or as specific as a goal, or a physiological and psychological concept (Bailey and Claus, 1975, pp. 109–10; Johnson et al., 1980, p. 102);
3. evaluation may not solely be the function of one nurse, but may be shared with another nurse and in some situations may be handled by a case conference (Kron, 1966, pp. 142–3);
4. the patient's views are important to the nurse-evaluator (McCarthy, 1981);
5. evaluation is an important way of judging the effectiveness of a problem-solving strategy (Kron, 1966, p. 60);

6. evaluation is used to check other phases, and to adjust those which are not functioning effectively (Kron, 1966, p. 60; Pont, 1986). It has a particularly strong association with implementation (Vitale et al., 1978);
7. evaluation is an important means of identifying problems (Johnson et al., 1980, pp. 97–102; Lauri, 1982);
8. evaluation may be a less important phase in problem solving than generally realised (Frederickson and Mayer, 1977, p. 1169; de la Cuesta, 1983; Waters, 1986). Informants made fewer comments on evaluation than any other phase.

Aspects of evaluation for which there is less or no particular support in the literature include:

1. the frequency of the evaluation is judged to be important and depends on the context of the situation;
2. relatives' views are considered important in the evaluation phase.

Summary

The qualitative analysis of the interview transcripts has produced a wealth of empirical data about the five specific phases of problem-solving in nursing. The findings in this chapter generally agree with those arising from the quantitative analysis in Chapter 6, and provide much more detail.

When considered together, Chapters 6 and 7 contribute to the theory of clinical problem-solving in nursing by:

1. confirming, by empirical study, many points in the literature derived from previously speculative statements on nursing problem-solving;
2. developing existing knowledge and raising awareness of important clinical processes in nursing;
3. questioning some problem-solving issues seemingly accepted in the nursing problem-solving literature;
4. providing some new and important insights about nursing problem-solving which warrant further research.

In the next chapter, the findings from this study will be used to develop a theory of nursing problem-solving. Aspects of the theory will then be compared with general theories and those specific to medical, managerial and educational problem-solving. The implications for nursing education and practice will also be discussed along with suggestions for further research.

8

Conclusions and Implications for Nursing

As pointed out in Chapter 5, the aim of this research was to contribute to the theory of problem-solving processes in nursing by systematic empirical study. The principal objectives were: (1) to investigate in depth the perceptions and understanding of nursing problem-solving demonstrated by experienced, newly qualified and learner nurses; (2) to develop a cognate theory of problem-solving in nursing; and (3) compare the emergent theory with other general theories and accounts of problem-solving in the literature of nursing and allied professions.

Perceptions and understanding of problem-solving

Protocol analysis of 116 interviews with informants focusing on five to seven vignettes on clinical problem-solving provided a rich source of data which have been analysed quantitatively in Chapter 6 and qualitatively in Chapter 7.

A number of striking points arise from the analysis of recognition or non-recognition of phases in Chapter 6.

1. Generally, the problem-solving phases were quite well identified by informants, even though the actual words 'problem identification', 'problem assessment', 'planning', 'implementation' and 'evaluation' were carefully avoided in the text of the vignettes (see Chapter 5, p. 47 for an explanation). An analysis of Figures 6.1–6.5 shows that:
   (a) in total, 51 per cent of the informants mentioned problem identification, although there were differences in recognition and non-recognition across the vignettes (see Figure 6.1);
   (b) problem assessment was recognised by 71 per cent of informants and, with the exception of Vignette 6, a majority discussed the phase in each case (see Figure 6.2);
   (c) 55 per cent of informants recognised planning, but the numbers who discussed the phase only reached a majority when this phase was actually included in the vignettes (see Figure 6.3);

(d) the largest proportion of informants (87 per cent) commented on implementation, and the number recognising the phase was statistically significant in each case (see Figure 6.4);

(e) 44 per cent mentioned evaluation, and as in the case of problem identification, there were differences in recognition and non-recognition across the vignettes (see Figure 6.5);

2. On the whole, there was less discussion when a problem-solving phase was omitted from a vignette than when a phase was included. Some phases were quite often not recognised, and there are some interesting and important variations in recognition and non-recognition. For example:

(a) problem assessment was missing in Vignettes 2 and 3, but as we can see from Figure 6.2, a total of 71 per cent of the informants commented on assessment when discussing these two vignettes;

(b) planning was omitted from Vignettes 3 and 7, but an inspection of Figure 6.3 shows that only 25 per cent mentioned it when discussing these two vignettes;

(c) implementation was missing in Vignette 5, and we can see from Figure 6.4 that 79 per cent mentioned it when discussing that vignette;

(d) evaluation was omitted from Vignettes 4 and 6, and Figure 6.5 shows that only 21 per cent mentioned it when discussing these two vignettes.

Problem identification cannot be analysed in this way because it was included in all the vignettes.

It is evident that assessment and implementation attracted more comment than identification, planning and evaluation. Indeed, sometimes the strength of comment on each of the former two phases exceeded comment on each of the latter three phases even when assessment and implementation were missing from the vignettes. For example, 84 per cent of the informants discussed problem assessment in Vignette 3 even when the phase was missing, against 55 per cent and 41 per cent who commented on problem identification and evaluation respectively when they were included. Likewise, 79 per cent mentioned implementation even when it was omitted from Vignette 5, which is a higher proportion than those who discussed problem identification (33 per cent) and evaluation (68 per cent) when the two phases were present.

3. As we have seen from the discussion of informants' pathway through the vignettes (pp. 66–9), their thinking process was not always systematic, an issue also raised by critics of the stages model theory (e.g. Forehand, 1966, p. 31). However, this could mean that informants were indeed following a stages model, but were using it flexibly, at least

in the reflective activities analysed. On the other hand, their problem-solving behaviour could perhaps be analysed in terms of the information-processing system theory.

4. Recognition or non-recognition of phases surprisingly was not strongly dependent on experience. There did not appear to be a relationship between nursing experience and the recognition or non-recognition of phases (see Table 6.2). This finding is also supported by evidence from Table 7.1, which shows that learner nurses were generally well represented among the contributors to the discussion of each category of response. This runs counter to the views of some writers (e.g. McCarthy, 1981; Carnevali et al., 1984, p. 40; Corcoran, 1986) who attach importance to the relationship between clinical experience and problem-solving performance. This is one aspect of problem-solving which requires further study.

The findings from Chapter 6 have provided new insights about clinical problem-solving in nursing, but some of the evidence is inconclusive. For example, the statistical analysis of recognition and non-recognition of phases, which underpins Chapter 6, revealed differences which were not always statistically significant, or sometimes showed a reversal of order between recognition and non-recognition in different vignettes. The implications of some of these findings are discussed later in this chapter.

The qualitative analysis in Chapter 7 provided a wealth of information about nurses' perceptions and understanding of problem solving. However, only those issues that attracted comment from at least five informants have been included (p. 71). The findings largely support the theoretical and empirical literature on nursing problem-solving. Sometimes, however, there was disagreement between the present findings and views expressed elsewhere, and occasionally new issues emerged which the researcher could not identify in the literature. In the section that follows, findings in the present research which support the literature are discussed first, followed by those which question literature statements and new issues.

Findings that support the literature

With regard to problem identification, there is support from the findings in this study for the views of Bailey and Claus (1975, p. 21) that timely and accurate recognition of problems is important to the patient's welfare. Johnson et al.'s (1980, p. 47) suggestion that problems can be identified by several means, is also supported. The view of some writers that problems are usually classified in some way, for example, as actual or potential problems as explained by Roper et al. (1983, p. 10), also gains support.

Concerning assessment, there is agreement with Bailey and Claus (1975, p. 21) and Lauri (1982) that an accurate and timely problem assessment is important to successful problem-solving, particularly when the nurse includes the patient and others in the assessment process. Some informants said that assessment is at least a two-stage procedure in which additional problems may be recognised and both old and new problems explored, in accordance with Johnson et al. (1980, p. 56) and Vitale et al. (1978, p. 38). Assessment was generally felt to be weak when insufficient data were collected, or when data were left uncorroborated or unclassified, points also raised by Aspinall (1976) and Corcoran (1986).

With reference to planning, the claim by Johnson et al. (1980, p. 144) that this stage focuses on the problems and related data arising from the problem identification and assessment stages is supported in this study. The subsequent goals and nursing interventions in the plan are usually prioritised in some way; for example, in line with the way related problems were ordered, as suggested by Vitale et al. (1978, p. 8). Also, the quality of the problem-solving process was felt to be improved when the patient was involved in the planning and implementation phases (Vitale et al., 1978, p. 8).

Nursing interventions were generally related to the plan, but there were occasions when an informant attempted to solve a problem without reference to the plan, and these actions seemed to be guided by experience, as suggested by Miller (1984). Informants agreed with Vitale et al. (1978, p. 83) that the timing of interventions was important. The educational benefit of the implementation phase for learner nurses, and the importance of accurate recording of information, was acknowledged by informants in this research, as they were by Priestley et al. (1979, p. 70) and Kron (1966, p. 65), respectively.

The finding that some nurses use the terms evaluation and assessment synonymously when discussing evaluation confirms findings by Vitale et al. (1978, p. 85). As explained by Kron (1966, p. 60), the main function of evaluation is to judge the effectiveness of nursing interventions and to adjust actions which appear not to be working is supported. It was noted that the evaluator may focus on several criteria (Bailey and Claus, 1975, p. 109), and that evaluation is not the sole province of the nurse (Kron, 1966, p. 142), for it may need to involve the patient and other health professionals. However, the suspicion of some writers (Frederickson and Mayer, 1977, p. 1169; de la Cuesta, 1983; Waters, 1986), that evaluation is perceived to be a less important stage than other stages in the problem-solving process, is confirmed in this study.

Findings that have only limited support in the literature

Some findings question problem-solving issues seemingly accepted in the nursing problem-solving literature. Planning was generally given less attention by informants in this study than many writers, (e.g. Hardy and Engel, 1987) say it deserves. The view of Johnson et al. (1980, p. 78), that the medical model provides an acceptable framework for the nursing plan, was denigrated by some informants, probably in protection of nursing autonomy. Indeed, the basis for nursing interventions in this study seemed much broader than the views of some writers; for example, it was said that interventions may sometimes be experience-based as well as goal-based.

New issues

Some aspects of problem-solving were raised by informants for which little or no reference could be found in the literature. For example, some informants felt in the problem identification phase that some problems would need to be confirmed with evidence from another source. Also informants attached importance to the relationship between the frequency of evaluation and the context of the situation and placed more emphasis on the value of involving the patient's relatives in the evaluation process than was apparent from the literature. The implications of these new issues are discussed later.

A theory of problem-solving in nursing

We can see from the preceding discussion that there are a number of findings in this research which lend support to a stages model theory of clinical problem-solving in nursing.

First, the phase model generally appeared to be understood by all types of nurse in this study. Without prompting, informants, in their discussion of the vignettes, used key vocabulary and phrases associated with stages models of problem-solving. Detailed examples of the use of the key words 'problem identification', 'assessment', 'implementation' and 'evaluation' can be seen in the quotations in Chapter 7. For example, a sister, commenting on Vignette 2, said: 'The learner nurse *identified the problem* and the sister *planned* the care.' On another occasion, a teacher remarked that the sister 'had sat down and talked to him [the patient] about his condition, so she has gone through a process of factual *assessment* . . .' The use of key words was not limited to the more senior nurses; a learner nurse, for example, noted that 'it doesn't actually say that the nursing care was *evaluated* or updated . . .'

Second, as we saw above, informants discussed individual phases of problem-solving even when a phase, notably problem assessment and implementation, was deliberately omitted from the vignette (see Figures 6.2, and 6.4, respectively). The instances in which merely a minority of informants discussed a phase, as in the case of planning in Vignettes 3 and 7, and evaluation in Vignettes 4 and 6 (see Figures 6.3 and 6.5, respectively) do not necessarily refute the argument that nurses are following a stages model in nursing. Rather, these findings extend our insights into the problem-solving process, in that some nurses seem to concentrate on the 'doing' aspects of nursing (implementation) at the expense of the analytical processes associated with planning and evaluation.

Third, informants sometimes made statements about specific phases with reference to other named, discrete phases of problem-solving in a logical way. For example, some informants referred to the assessment data when discussing the planning phase, e.g. Category 18 (p. 87), 'relationship between planning and assessment'. The logical connection between phases was further illustrated when some informants linked their statements about the 'goal' and 'action' elements when discussing the planning and implementation phases, for example, see Category 33, 'role of planning/goals' (p. 98). Likewise, when discussing evaluation, informants sometimes considered other phases, as in the case of Category 47, 'a means of judging the plan or action' (p. 105).

Finally, the qualitative analysis has revealed much support for issues discussed in the literature whose writers implicitly, and sometimes explicitly support a stages model. Examples can be seen in the summaries of each phase within Chapter 7, and in the earlier discussion in this chapter.

On the whole, it is felt that the informants' level of discussion would not have been possible without an implicit if not explicit understanding of a stages model, together with some experience of applying the model to everyday work.

However, three caveats need to be added regarding the evidence given here for a stages model theory in nursing. First, it must be remembered that this model was used in the design of the vignettes. Although the key words 'problem identification', 'problem assessment', 'planning', 'implementation' and 'evaluation' were deliberately not included in the text of the vignettes, the implicit stages model framework may have influenced informants' thinking. Second, informants were commenting on second-hand accounts of clinical problem solving. As pointed out in Chapter 5 (p. 57), the vignettes may have prompted informants to discuss problem-solving issues not normally considered, and may not have allowed them free rein in their discussion. Third, protocol analysis, as a means of analysing and interpreting a person's thinking and understanding of the problem-solving process, has some weaknesses as we saw in Chapter 5 (p. 45).

A comparison with problem-solving in allied professions

The medical, managerial and educational literature on problem-solving was discussed in Chapter 4. It is felt that a comparison of the main theoretical issues arising from Chapter 4 with the emergent theory from this research would further clarify the problem-solving process in nursing.

One outcome of the literature review was that medical diagnosis is considered to be a problem-solving process in itself, and the patient management process is another, separate problem-solving process. That is, as Palva (1974) and McGuire (1985) suggest, the diagnostic reasoning approach to problem-solving appears to be simply a labelling process. Conversely, some nurses, as described in this study and in supporting literature, appear to use a more complete process of problem-solving than merely identifying the problem. That is, some appear to go on to plan, implement and evaluate nursing interventions to overcome the problem.

In the diagnostic problem-solving process, the act of diagnosis can be compared with the problem identification phase in some nursing situations (Tanner, 1987). Currently, this is not true of nursing in the United Kingdom, because the diagnosis of nursing problems is not commonly taught or practised in this country. However, it is felt by some researchers that nurses will attend more to diagnostic reasoning research in the future because of its superiority over the stages model. Its superiority allegedly arises from its subtler means of describing the detailed cognitive processes involved in solving problems. The potential benefits which this more detailed understanding bestows upon nurse education are being recognised.

It is believed to be only a matter of time before the techniques of diagnostic reasoning research are also applied to the planning, implementing and evaluation processes (Carnevali et al., 1984, pp. 237–8). An argument for undertaking more research into diagnostic problem-solving, as we have seen in Chapter 3 (p. 15), is that the diagnostic reasoning approach better explains the differences between expert and novice nurse problem solvers (Tanner et al., 1987).

It seemed that more of the medical problem-solving literature was empirically-based than was the case in the nursing literature. This may simply be a result of research being more established in medical education and practice than is the case in nursing.

Interestingly, Simon et al. (1987, p. 24) believe that our understanding of the information-processing approach to problem-solving in management is also felt to be lacking, owing to a dearth of empirical work. The stages models appear to be more popular in the management literature (as in nursing), and many of these stages models are very similar to those described in nursing, as are many of the sub-processes within each phase (Greenwood et al., 1983, pp. 15–21).

Problems in nursing (and medicine) tend to be human-related, whereas problems in management are generally resource-based. As we have seen, the type of problem can determine the problem-solving approach used by the manager (Greenwood et al., 1983), but the nurse managers in this study did not appear to let the problem type influence their strategies any more than other nurses' actions. Further research is needed to determine whether the characteristics of the problem are also important determinants in a nurse's problem-solving strategy.

Another issue in the management literature, which is not usually addressed in problem-solving literature of related disciplines, was Shone's (1974, pp. 23–4) recommendation that certain steps in one managerial stages model of problem-solving may be omitted to save time and improve efficiency. It will be recalled that some nurses did not apparently make use of one or more phases in their discussion of problem-solving, so Shone's recommendation may also apply to nursing. This is an issue also worthy of further research.

Other approaches to managerial problem-solving were discussed in the literature, but tended to include methods for specific management situations; for example, for dealing with conflict between management and employees (Margerison, 1974, pp. 14–33). It is unusual to find purpose-designed methods of problem-solving for specific situations in the nursing literature. Perhaps in the light of the present research, where nurses' problem-solving seems to be related to the context of the problem, more consideration should be given to testing a variety of problem-solving strategies in different contexts.

Problem-solving in educational settings shares common ground with nursing and medicine in that it has a strong inter-personal element (Hill, 1979). A major difference between education and the other disciplines is that the research is divided into two distinct categories: (1) problem-solving as a means of facilitating learning; and (2) research into the cognitive processes of problem-solving for the purpose of increasing understanding. In the case of research designed to facilitate learning using problem-solving as a teaching and learning strategy, discussion is mostly about the practical problems of teaching and learning as highlighted by Schmuck et al. (1966). The stages models used here are comparable to nursing stages models and, to a lesser extent, management models too (Schmuck et al., 1966). In these disciplines, the emphasis is on problem recognition, problem analysis, action and evaluation.

The second type of educational problem-solving research is that into the cognitive processes of problem-solving (Garrett, 1986). It is the information-processing system theory which is attracting interest and gaining importance here (Tuma and Reif, 1980). An active area of educational research is on the differences between the problem-solving ability of novices compared with experts (Stewart, 1985). This is an aspect which is also researched in medicine, management and nursing in North America, but not so much in nursing in the United Kingdom, probably because of the paucity of problem-solving research in this country to date. However, the issue of novice and expert nursing is likely to become important in the United Kingdom with the development of Project 2000 (UKCC, 1985) and PREPP (Post-Registration Education and Practice Project) (UKCC, 1990).

As we have seen in Chapter 4 (p. 39), the educational literature has a unique feature in the form of the independent stance taken by Schön (1987). The model of educational problem-solving described by him is similar to the information-processing system theory. Schön emphasises the diagnostic process in his description of problem-solving which, as we have seen, is also felt to be important in some explanations of medical problem-solving (Elstein et al., 1978) and nursing problem-solving in North America (Tanner et al., 1987). It is likely that Schön's educational model will influence other disciplines including nursing in the United Kingdom. Indeed, Champion (1988) reported an experimental nursing curriculum in this country which is strongly influenced by the work of Schön.

There appears to be one main difference and one main similarity between the four professional disciplines discussed in this research. The difference is the way medicine favours the information-processing system theory as a means of describing and exploring medical problem-solving in contrast to the other three, which tend to concentrate on stages models. Notwithstanding the independent stance of medicine, the stages models of problem-solving do seem to have a universal quality across the disciplines. There are, however, some differences in the sub-processes within each of the stages.

Implications of the study and recommendations for further research

This chapter has summarised some important findings which have implications for current nursing theory and practice, or raise questions needing further study. Some of these are as follows:

1. Because the findings from this research lend support to a stages model theory of clinical problem-solving, the continued use of this model in nursing practice seems sensible. But there are a number of concerns about the model; for example, as we have seen, the failure of many nurses to comment on what were hitherto considered to be necessary stages in

clinical problem-solving (especially problem identification, planning and evaluation) is surprising and perhaps worrying, and requires additional study.

Furthermore, the relationship between problem identification and assessment is not yet entirely clear. Some nurses in this study used identified problems to assist the assessment, whilst others listed the problems as a product of an assessment based on, for example, a model of living (Roper et al., 1983). Encouragement in using assessment to identify problems may cause difficulties for nurses who structure the assessment process according to recognised problems. It is felt, therefore, that nurse teachers and practitioners need to recognise related differences in nurses' thinking.

The high degree of attention given to implementation at the possible expense of planning and evaluation needs explaining. Indeed, the role of evaluation in nursing problem-solving, from both the general literature and specific nursing problem-solving literature (see the high citation count for evaluation in Table 2.2), has been rendered problematic by this research. It seems that this stage has an important part to play in nursing problem-solving, yet the relative unimportance attached to evaluation by the majority of nurses in the sample, when reviewing accounts of problem-solving, is puzzling. These findings tend to confirm the results of de la Cuesta's (1983) and Waters' (1986) research. Has the apparent lack of importance arisen because of insufficient attention to evaluation in nurse education or has it arisen because nurses use some other mechanism(s) to judge the success of nursing interventions? Or again, could it be that nurses simply concentrate on the 'doing' aspects of nursing at the expense of the analytical processes of problem-solving? These questions cannot yet be fully answered and need further study.

There are appreciable similarities between the phase model emergent in the present study and some contemporary descriptions of the nursing process, which is commonly described as one form of problem-solving. But there is evidence in this study that a general stages model may not always explain how nurses think, owing to variations in perceptions and understanding of problem-solving demonstrated in the interviews. This finding is perhaps not surprising since nurses (1) are taught by many different teachers; (2) work and gain experience in a variety of clinical settings; (3) are supervised by different managers; and (4) are exposed to a variety of nursing literature. In short, the variety of nursing education and practical experiences combine to create the unique practitioner.

If nurses bring different problem-solving styles to their jobs and educational programmes, the adherence to a rigidly linear four- or five-stage model may be alien to some nurses' thinking. Managers and teachers, therefore, may need to be more flexible in their approaches to the practice and teaching of nursing. There may be a need to introduce a more adaptable method of problem-solving in which nurses may add or remove stages according to their experience and/or the context of the problem.

There is little evidence to date that these individual problem-solving styles are effective, an issue that may have repercussions upon the quality of nursing care. There is a clear, need, therefore, to examine the relationship between the clinical problem-solving process and nursing outcome. In a similar vein, the nurses' Code of Professional Conduct (UKCC, 1984) has an important bearing upon an individual's problem-solving ability, in that each practitioner will be held accountable for his or her professional practice.

2. Some of the findings in this study which have little or no mention in the literature need to be recognised by nurses, and perhaps ought to be included in the nursing curriculum. First, confirming nursing problems with corroborative evidence was felt to be important by some informants. This suggests that an appropriate prompt could be added to the nursing assessment sheet reminding the nurse to seek further evidence. Second, the informants' perceived frequency of evaluation was related to the context of the problem. Not only does this indicate that evaluation is important, but also that there may be a significant sub-process to be considered when teaching and practising evaluation. Third, some prominence was given to the involvement of the patient's relatives in the evaluation process by informants in this study. Indeed, the relative's long-standing knowledge of the patient's circumstances may provide an important insight and an additional indicator for judging the effectiveness of nursing care.

3. The finding that some nurses demonstrated a non-linear approach when written accounts of problem-solving were analysed and interpreted was a little surprising; though it must be pointed out that reflecting and speaking about problem-solving scenarios is not the same as enacting problem-solving. However, if nurses do use a non-linear approach in their clinical work, there may be a need, as explained earlier, to adopt a more flexible approach to practical problem-solving in nursing education, or to consider other problem-solving theories such as the information-processing and diagnostic reasoning approaches.

Since this research has not investigated the validity of the information-processing system theory of problem-solving, clearly there is now a need to plan and implement further work to evaluate the importance of this under-researched theory in nursing. Additional study would benefit nursing in the United Kingdom in two ways: first, by adding to what is known about nurses' thinking; and second, by providing a sounder theoretical base to nursing education and practice.

4. There is also a need to examine clinical problem-solving using research methods different from the ones employed in the present research. For example, problem-solving could also be investigated using a

method more closely related, both in time and approach, to the actual process of clinical problem-solving. The critical incident technique might be a possible method of investigation. A variant of this technique would be to interview practitioners immediately after participating in an unrehearsed problem-solving episode on the ward (but not necessarily seen as critical by the practitioner), incorporating a protocol analysis similar to that used in this study.

Another method of investigation might be to use computer-based problem-solving simulations. These would present the user with pre-prepared clinical problem-solving situations, allowing selection of a problem-solving strategy, the process of which would be recorded by the computer for later analysis. An important spin-off would be the incorporation of the program in a computer-assisted learning package for less-experienced nurses.

5. Computers could have other roles too in the field of problem-solving research. For example, one useful (but peripheral) outcome from this study was the development of a prototype computer program written specifically for the qualitative analysis of interview transcripts as described in Chapter 5 (p. 55). The program has been extensively tested, and although no rigorous measurements have been made, it is estimated that the speed of data analysis has been increased by approximately a factor of 10 when compared with a manual analysis. Already, the program has proved beneficial in two other major research projects, and it has generated considerable interest following publication (Hurst et al., 1989). Development and testing of the program is continuing and further publications are planned.

6. The differences between novice and expert nurse problem-solvers have been examined briefly in this thesis. Developments in basic and post-basic nursing education programmes, with the stress placed on the 'knowledgeable practitioner', are increasingly likely to emphasise the importance of understanding novice and expert thinking and practice (Project 2000, UKCC, 1985; PREPP, UKCC, 1990). These developments may add further momentum to research into problem-solving, not least because outcomes may influence the teaching and practice of individualised patient care based on a problem-solving approach. It is important that both first-level and second-level nurses have opportunities to update themselves within this rapidly developing clinical approach via, for example, appropriate post-basic, in-service education courses.

7. The similarities and differences between the problem-solving process in nursing and that in medicine, management and education have been briefly explored. It is felt that much more can be learned by further comparative empirical studies, especially by investigating the wider implications of problem-solving behaviour peculiar to one discipline.

Further work as suggested above would certainly extend our knowledge and understanding of nursing problem-solving, a laudable endeavour in a period of significant change in nursing education and practice when the provision of high-quality patient care and the development of the nurse's professional skills are at the forefront of current debate.

References

Abdellah F G (1957) Methods of identifying covert aspects of nursing problems. *Nursing Research*, **6**: 4–23.

Ackoff R L (1978) *The Art of Problem Solving*. New York: Wiley.

Aggleton P and Chalmers H (1984) Models and theories. Defining the terms. *Nursing Times*, **80**, 36: 24–8.

Aggleton P and Chalmers H (1986) Nursing research, nursing theory and the nursing process. *Journal of Advanced Nursing*, **11**: 197–202.

Algie J and Foster W (1984) *The Priority Decision System*. London: Work Sciences Associates.

Ashworth P (1980) Nursing process. Problems and solutions. *Nursing Mirror*, **151**, 12: 34–7.

Ashworth P and Castledine G (1981) The way we teach . . . nursing – using the nursing process. *Medical Teacher*, **3**, 3: 87–91.

Aspinall M J (1976) Nursing diagnosis – the weak link. *Nursing Outlook*, **24**, 7: 433–7.

Attree M J (1982) *The Relationship between Creative Thinking and Problem Solving Ability in Student Nurses*. Unpublished MSc Thesis, University of Manchester.

Bailey J T and Claus K (1975) *Decision Making in Nursing*. London: Mosby.

Bale P (1984) The impact of organizational culture on approaches to organizational problem solving. *Organization Studies*, **5**, 1: 43–66.

Barker P (1987) Assembling the pieces. *Nursing Times*, **83**, 47: 67–8.

Barnett D (1985) Making your plans work. *Nursing Times*, **81**, 2: 24–7.

Barnett O (1984) Computer-based simulations and clinical problem solving. *Medical Informatics*, **9**, 3/4: 277–9.

Baron J (1989) *Thinking and Deciding*. Cambridge: Cambridge University Press.

Basford P, Balcombe K and Chakravarti J (1987) A goal-less draw. *Senior Nurse*, **6**, 5: 24–6.

Baumann A and Deber R (1986) *Rapid decision making by nurses: is decision analysis appropriate?* Proceedings of the International Nursing Research Conference, Edmonton, Canada.

Beeler J (1987) The nuts and bolts of decision making and problem solving. *Data Management*, **25**, 10: 23–5.

Berner E S (1984) Paradigms and problem solving: a literature review. *Journal of Medical Education*, **59**, August: 625–33.

Beswetherick M (1979) Staffing assignment: a review of past and current systems of nursing care delivery. *Canadian Nurse*, **75**, 5: 18–22.

Bloch D (1974) Some crucial terms in nursing. What do they really mean? *Nursing Outlook*, **22**, 11: 689–94.

Bloom B S, Englehart M D, Furst E J, Hill W H and Krathwol D (eds) (1956) *Taxonomy of Educational Objectives Handbook 1: Cognitive Domain*. London: Longman.

Boreham N C (1977) The use of case histories to assess nurses ability to solve clinical problems. *Journal of Advanced Nursing,* **2**: 57–66.

Boreham N C (1986) A model of efficiency in diagnostic problem solving: implications for the education of diagnosticians. *Instructional Science,* **15**: 191–211.

Boylan A (1982) Nursing at the crossroads – 2. The nursing process and the role of the registered nurse. *Nursing Times,* **78**, 35: 1443–4.

Brazell H and Mansfield J (1984) Tackling problems. *Health and Social Services Journal,* **94**, 4878: 23.

Breckman B (1986) Success by stages. *Senior Nurse,* **5**, 3: 14–16.

Brightman H S and Verhoeven P (1986) Running successful problem-solving groups (part 2). *Business,* **36**, 2: 15–23.

Brown G D, Kaluzny A and Feirman H (1981) *Towards Problem Solving: Options Analysis and Implementation.* Washington: Association of University Programs in Health Administration.

Buckenham M (1986) Patient's points of view. *Senior Nurse,* **4**, 3: 26–7.

Burton L (1979) Introduction. In C C Hill, *Problem Solving: Learning and Teaching an Annotated Bibliography.* London: Pinter.

Calderhead J (ed.) (1987) *Exploring Teachers' Thinking.* London: Cassell Educational.

Callin M and Ciliska D (1983) Revitalizing problem solving with triple jump. *Canadian Nurse,* **79**, 3: 41–4.

Carnevali D, Mitchell P, Woods N and Tanner C A (1984) *Diagnostic Reasoning in Nursing.* Philadelphia: Lipincott.

Carroll E (1988) The role of tacit knowledge in problem solving in the clinical setting. *Nurse Education Today,* **8**: 140–7.

Champion R (1988) Competent nurses? Reflective practitioner? *Pathways to Progress, Conference Proceedings.* The School of Nursing Studies, University of Wales, July.

Chapman C (1974) Nurse education. *Nursing Times,* **70**, 18: 660–2.

Chenitz W C and Swanson J M (1984) Surfacing nursing process: a method of generating nursing theory from practice. *Journal of Advanced Nursing,* **9**: 205–15.

Chi M T H and Glaser R. (1984) Problem-solving ability. In R J Sternberg (ed.) *Human Abilities an Information Processing Approach.* New York: Freeman.

Chrisof C (1939) The formulation and elaboration of thought-problems. *The American Journal of Psychology,* **LII**, 2: 161–85.

Clarke M (1978) Planning nursing care: recent past, present and future. *Nursing Times,* Occasional Papers, **74**, 5: 17–20.

Colightly C K (1981) *Creative Problem Solving for Health Care Professionals.* Maryland: Aspend.

Corcoran S (1986) Task complexity and nursing expertise as factors in decision making. *Nursing Research,* **35**, 2: 107–12.

Cormack D F S (1984) *The Research Process in Nursing.* Oxford: Blackwell Scientific Publications.

Cousins D (1986) Computer aided learning, computer literacy and the nurse tutor. *Conference Proceedings CBT '86.* Keele University, September.

Cox K and Ewan C (eds) (1982) *Medical Teacher.* London: Churchill Livingstone.

Crout E (1987) Nursing process. The management process. *Senior Nurse,* **6**, 5: 26–8.

Crow J (1980) *Effects of Preparation on Problem Solving.* London: Royal College of Nursing.

Darcy P T (1980) The nursing process – a base for all developments. *Nursing Times*, **76**, 20: 497–501.

Data Protection Registrar (1985) *The Data Protection Act 1984*. Wilmslow: HMSO.

Dawson M D (1956) Lectures versus problem solving in teaching elementary soil science. *Science Education*, **40**, 5: 395–404.

de la Cuesta C (1983) The nursing process: from development to implementation. *Journal of Advanced Nursing*, **8**: 365–71.

de Tornyay R (1970) *Strategies for Teaching Nursing*. London: John Wiley.

del Bueno D J (1983) Doing the right thing: nurses ability to make clinical decisions. *Nurse Educator*, **8**: 7–11.

Docking S and Neave J (1986) The challenge of change. *Senior Nurse*, **5**, 2: 26–8.

Draper P (1986) Any use for an American import? *Nursing Times*, **82**, 8: 37–9.

Duncan C P (1959) Recent research on problem solving, *Psychological Bulletin*, **56**: 397–429.

Eddy D M (1984) Variations in physician practice: the role of uncertainty. *Health Affairs*, **3**, 2: 74–89.

Eden C, Jones S and Sims D (1983) *Messing about in Problems: an Informal Structured Approach to their Identification and Management*. Oxford: Pergamon Press.

Egan G (1982) *The Skilled Helper*, 2nd edn. London: Brooks and Cale.

Elstein A S, Shulman L S and Sprafka S A (1978) *Medical Problem Solving. An Analysis of Clinical Reasoning*. Cambridge, Mass.: Harvard University Press.

Feightner J W, Barrows H S, Neufeld V R and Norman G (1977) General medicine. Solving problems: how does the family practitioner do it? *Canadian Family Physician*, **23**, 457: 67–71.

Field P A and Morse J (1985) *Nursing Research: The Application of Qualitative Approaches*. London: Croom Helm.

Filkins J (1986) Introducing change. *Nursing Times*, **82**, 7: 26–9.

Flanagan J C (1954) The critical incident technique. *Psychological Bulletin*, **51**, 4: 327–58.

Forehand G (1966) Epilogue: constructs and strategies from problem-solving research. In B Kleinmuntz (ed.) *Problem Solving: Research, Method, and Theory*. New York: John Wiley.

Foxhall G R (1986) Managerial orientations of adaptors and innovators. *Journal of Managerial Psychology*, **1**, 2: 24–7.

Frederickson K and Mayer G G (1977) Problem-solving skills: what effect does education have? *American Journal of Nursing*, **70**, July: 1167–9.

Frisbie D A (1983) Testing beyond the knowledge level. *Journal of Nursing Education*, **22**, 6: 228–31.

Frisbie D A (1984) Looking at teaching through the nursing process. *Journal of Nursing Education*, **23**, 9: 401–3.

Gagné R M (1966) Human problem solving: internal and external events. In B Kleinmuntz (ed.) *Problem Solving: Research, Method, and Theory*. New York: John Wiley.

Gagné R M (1967) *The Conditions of Learning*. New York: Holt Rinehart and Winston.

Garrett R M (1986) Problem solving in science education. *Studies in Science Education*, **13**: 70–95.

General Nursing Council for England and Wales (1977) *Training Syllabus: Register of Nurses*. London: General Nursing Council for England and Wales.

Geogopnilos B S (1986) *Organisational Structure, Problem Solving, and Effectiveness: A Comparative Study of Hospital Emergency Services*. San Francisco: Jossey-Bass.

Gillis J G (1983) Improve your creativity, problem solving and decision-making quotients. *Journal of Forms Management*, **8**, 3: 23–5.

Goble I W J (1981) Educating the professional nurse of tomorrow . . . today. *Nursing Times*, **77**, 17: 746–8.

Goor A and Sommerfield R E (1975) A comparison of problem-solving processes of creative and non-creative students. *Journal of Educational Psychology*, **67**, 4: 495–505.

Greaves F (1987) Learning the scientific method. *Senior Nurse*, **6**, 6: 23–4.

Green B (1966) Introduction: Current trends in problem solving. In B Kleinmuntz (ed.) *Problem Solving: Research, Method, and Theory*. New York: John Wiley.

Greeno J G (1978) Nature of problem-solving abilities. In W K Estes (ed.) *Handbook of Learning and Cognitive Processes*. New Jersey: Lawrence Erlbaum Associates.

Greeno J G (1980) Trends in the theory of knowledge for problem solving. In D T Tuma and F Reif (eds) *Problem Solving and Education: Issues in Teaching and Research*. New Jersey: Lawrence Erlbaum Associates.

Greenwood N, Clark P, Johnston I, Dyson T and Kershaw G (1983) *Problem-Solving Matters. Case Studies in British Hospital Administration*. London: Institute of Health Service Administrators.

Guilford J P (1959) *Personality*. New York: McGraw-Hill.

Hammond K R (1966) Clinical inference in nursing II. A psychologist's view. *Nursing Research*, **15**, 1: 27–38.

Harasym P H, Alexander F, Baumber J S, Bryant H, Fundytus D, MacPhail I, Preshaw R, Sosnowski M, Watanabe M and Wyse G (1979) The underlying structure of clinical problem solving: process or content? *Proceedings of the Eighteenth Annual Conference on Research in Medical Education*.

Hardy L and Engel J (1987) The search for professionalism. *Nursing Times*, **83**, 15: 37–9.

Harris P and Hingley P (1987) *Manual of the Job Stress Indicator*. Unpublished, Bristol Polytechnic.

Harrison S, Haywood S and Fussell C (1984) Problems and solutions: the perceptions of NHS managers. *Hospital and Health Service Review*, **80**, 4: 185–8.

Hayes J R (1966) Memory, goals and problem solving. In B Kleinmuntz (ed.) *Problem Solving: Research, Method, and Theory*. New York: John Wiley.

HCEA (Health Care Education Associates) (1987) *Group Leadership Skills for Nurse Managers*. Washington: C V Mosby.

Hefferin E A and Hunter R E (1975) Nursing assessment and care plan statements. *Nursing Research*, **24**, 5: 360–6.

Helfer R E and Slater C H (1971) Measuring the process of solving clinical diagnostic problems. *British Journal of Medical Education*, **5**: 48–52.

Henderson V (1982) The nursing process – is the title right? *Journal of Advanced Nursing*, **7**: 103–9.

Hill C C (ed.) (1979) *Problem Solving: Learning and Teaching an Annotated Bibliography*. London: Pinter.

Holbert C M and Abraham C (1988) Reflections on teaching generic thinking and problem solving. *Nurse Educator*, **13**, 2: 23–7.

Hollingworth S (1985) *Preparation for Change. Preparing Nurse Tutors in Initial Training for a Change to Nursing Process*. London: Royal College of Nursing.

Hollingworth S (1986) The nursing process: implications for curriculum planning. *Journal of Advanced Nursing*, **11**: 211–16.

Holm K and Llewellyn J G (1986) *Nursing Research for Nursing Practice*. London: W B Saunders.

Holzemer W L (1986) The structure of problem solving in simulations. *Nursing Research*, **35**, 4: 231–6.

Huckabay L M D (1980) *Conditions of Learning and Instruction in Nursing: Modularised*. London: Mosby.

Hudkins B B (1966) *Problem Solving in the Classroom*. New York: Macmillan.

Hurst K, Dean A and Trickey S (1989) Modern approaches to qualitative research in nursing. *Nursing Times*, **85**, 28: 59.

Hutchins D (1985) *Quality Circles Handbook*. London: Pitman.

Isenberg D J (1986) Thinking and managing: a verbal protocol analysis of managerial problem solving. *Academy of Management Journal*, **29**, 4: 775–88.

Itano J K (1989) A comparison of the clinical judgement process in experienced registered nurses and student nurses. *Journal of Nursing Education*, **28**, 3: 120–6.

Johnson D (1984) A team approach to care. *Nursing Times*, **80**, 50: 50–1.

Johnson D M (1944) A modern account of problem solving. *Psychological Bulletin*, **41**, 4: 201–29.

Johnson D M (1955) *The Psychology of Thought and Judgement*. New York: Harper.

Johnson M M, Davis M L C and Lawbaugh A M (1980) *Problem Solving in Nursing Practice*, 3rd edn. Iowa: William C Brown.

Johnson P E, Moller J H and Bass G M (1975) Analysis of expert diagnosis of a computer simulation of clinical heart disease. *Journal of Medical Education*, **50**, 5: 466–70.

Jones B M (1986) *Problem Solving Examples in NHS Finance*. London: Institute of Health Service Management.

Jones J (1988) Clinical reasoning in nursing. *Journal of Advanced Nursing*, **13**: 185–92.

Jones J (1989) The verbal protocol: a research technique for nursing. *Journal of Advanced Nursing*, **14**: 1062–70.

Jones M and Sado M (1985) Circles of wisdom. *Nursing Mirror*, **161**, 3: s12–s13.

Joorabchi B (1981) How to . . . construct problem-solving MCQ's. *Medical Teacher*, **3**, 1: 9–13.

Kahney H (1986) *Problem Solving: a Cognitive Approach*. Milton Keynes: Open University Press.

Kaufmann R (1982) *Identifying and Solving Problems: a Systems Approach*, 3rd edn. California: University Associates Inc.

Kelly K (1966) An approach to the study of clinical inference in nursing: part 3 utilisation of the 'lens model' method to the study of the inferential process of the nurse. *Nursing Research*, **13**: 320.

Kendler H H (1961) Problems in problem solving research. In W Dennier (ed.) *Current Trends in Psychological Theory*. Pittsburgh: University of Pittsburgh Press.

Kershaw B (1987) Education for care. *Senior Nurse*, **6**, 6: 28–9.

King E C (1983) Humanistic education: theory and teaching strategies. *Nurse Educator*, **8**, 4: 39–42.

Kissinger J and Munjas B A (1981) Nursing process, student attributes and teaching methodologies. *Nursing Research*, **30**, 4: 242–6.

Kleinmuntz B (ed.) (1966) *Problem Solving: Research, Method, and Theory*. New York: John Wiley.

Kron T (1966) *Nursing Team Leadership*, 2nd edn. Philadelphia: W B Saunders.

Larkin J H (1980) Teaching problem solving in physics: the psychological laboratory and the practical classroom. In D T Tuma and F Reif (eds) (1980) *Problem Solving and Education: Issues in Teaching and Research*. New Jersey: Lawrence Erlbaum Associates.

128   Problem-solving in Nursing Practice

Larson L (1986) Improvement management deelopment through small problem-solving groups. *Journal of Management Development,* **5**, 2: 15–26.

Lauri S (1982) Development of the nursing process through action research. *Journal of Advanced Nursing,* **7**: 301–7.

Lawrence P (1984) *Management in Action.* London: Routledge & Kegan Paul.

Leigh A (1984) *Decisions, Decisions: a Practical Management Guide to Problem Solving and Decision Making.* Aldershot: Gower.

Lewis L (1976) *Planning Patient Care: Foundation of Nursing Series.* Massachusetts: Little, Brown.

Lindblom C E and Cohen D K (1979) *Usable Knowledge: Social Science and Social Problem Solving.* New Haven: Yale University Press.

Margerison C J (1974) *Managerial Problem Solving.* London: McGraw-Hill.

Marks-Maran D (1983) Can nurses diagnose? *Nursing Times,* **79**, 4: 68–9.

Marriner-Tomey A (1988) *Guide to Nursing Management,* 3rd edn. St Louis: Mosby.

Mayers M C (1972) *A Systematic Approach to the Nursing Care Plan.* New York: Appleton-Century-Crofts.

McCarthy M M (1981) The nursing process: application of current thinking in clinical problem solving. *Journal of Advanced Nursing,* **6**: 173–7.

McFarland G K, Skipton L H and Morris M M (1984) *Nursing Leadership and Management Contemporary Strategies.* Chichester: Wiley.

McGuire C H (1985) Medical problem solving: a critique of the literature. *Journal of Medical Education,* **60**, August: 587–95.

Merrifield P R, Guilford J P, Christensen P R and Frick J W (1962) The role of intellectual factors in problem solving. *Psychological Monographs: General and Applied,* **76**, 10, Whole No. 529: 1–21.

Miller A F (1984) Nursing process and patient care. *Nursing Times,* Occasional Paper, **8**, 13: 56–8.

Miller A F (1985) Right for the job? *Nursing Times,* **81**, 25: 44–6.

Montague S E (1982) Problems encountered in developing an appropriate strategy to investigate theoretical knowledge used by nurses as basis for clinical practice. In S Harrison (ed.) (1982) *Royal College of Nursing Annual Research Conference Number 23.* London: Royal College of Nursing.

Munro M F (1982) Analysis of problem solving strategies in nursing using written simulations of clinical situations. In M S Henderson (ed.) *Recent Advances in Nurse Education.* London: Churchill Livingstone.

Neufeld V R, Norman G R, Feightner J W and Burrows H S (1981) Clinical problem solving by medical students: a cross-sectional and longitudinal analysis. *Medical Education,* **15**: 315–22.

Newell A and Simon H A (1972) *Human Problem Solving.* New Jersey: Prentice-Hall.

Palva I P (1974) Measuring clinical problem solving. *British Journal of Medical Education,* **8**: 52–6.

Pardue S F (1987) Decision-making skills and critical thinking ability among associate degree, diploma, baccalaureate, and master's-prepared nurses. *Journal of Nursing Education,* **26**, 9: 354–61.

Phillips L R and Rempusheski V F (1985) A decision-making model for diagnosing and intervening in elderly abuse and neglect. *Nursing Research,* **34**, 3: 134–9.

Phillips R L, Posner B and Walker D (1985) A strategy for inter-unit problem solving. *Health Care Management Review,* **10**, 1: 53–9.

Polit F D and Hungler P B (1987) *Nursing Research. Principles and Methods,* 2nd edn. Philadelphia: J B Lippincott.

Polson P G and Jeffries R (1982) Problem solving as search and understanding. In R J Sternberg (ed.) *Advances in the Psychology of Human Intelligence.* New Jersey: Lawrence Erlbaum Associates.

Polya G (1963) *How to Solve it.* New Jersey: Princeton University Press.

Pont M (1986) Nursing practice. Last but not least. *Nursing Times,* **82**, 41: 54–5.

Priestley P, McGuire J, Flegg D, Hemsley V and Welham D (1979) *Social Skills and Personal Problem Solving: a Handbook of Methods.* London: Social Science Paperbacks, Tavistock.

Putzier D, Tanner C A, Westfall U E and Padrick K P (1986) Verbal protocol analysis: a new approach to the study of diagnostic reasoning in nurses. *Proceedings of the International Nursing Research Conference.* Edmonton, Canada.

Rakich J S, Longest B B and Darr K (1985) *Managing Health Services Organizations.* Philadelphia: Saunders.

Rawlinson J G (1981) *Introduction to Creative Thinking and Brain-storming.* London: British Institute of Management.

Rhodes B (1984) *An Investigation Into the Usefulness of a Theoretical Decision-Making Model of Nursing.* Unpublished PhD Thesis, University of Leeds.

Richardson J and Bennett B (1984) Applying learning techniques to on-the-job development (part 2). *Journal of European Industrial Training,* **8**, 3: 5–10.

Rickards T (1985) *Stimulating Innovation: A Systems Approach.* London: Pinter.

Riehl J P and Roy C (1980) *Conceptual Models for Nursing Practice,* 2nd edn. New York: Appleton-Century-Crofts.

Rodgers J A (1976) Today's preparation for tomorrow's practice: the Leham Nursing Programme. *Journal of Advanced Nursing,* **1**: 311–22.

Roper N, Logan W and Tierney A (eds) (1983) *Using a Model for Nursing.* Edinburgh: Churchill Livingstone.

Schön D A (1987) *Educating the Reflective Practitioner.* San Francisco: Jossey-Bass.

Schmieding N J (1987) Problematic situations in nursing: analysis of Orlando's theory based on Dewey's theory of inquiry. *Journal of Advanced Nursing,* **12**: 431–40.

Schmuck R, Chester M and Lippitt R (1966) *Problem Solving to Improve Classroom Learning.* Chicago: Science Research Associate.

Sculco C D (1978) Development of a taxonomy for the nursing process. *Journal of Nursing Education,* **17**, 6: 40–8.

Sharples S (1987) DRG's and computing. *British Journal of Health Computing,* **4**, 5: 27–31.

Sheaf R (1985) Two uses for a problem-solving exercise. *Health Service Manpower Review,* **11**, 2: 17–21.

Shone K J (1974) *Problem Solving for Managers.* London: Collins.

Simon H A (1975) The functional equivalence of problem solving skills. *Cognitive Psychology,* **7**: 268–88.

Simon H A and Hayes J R (1985) Information processing theories of human problem solving. In A M Aitkenhead and J M Slack (eds) *Issues in Cognitive Modelling.* New Jersey: Lawrence Erlbaum Associates.

Simon H A, Dantzig G B, Hogarth R, Plott C R, Raiffa H, Schelling T C, Shepsie K A, Thaller R, Tversky A and Winter S (1987) Decision making and problem solving. *Interfaces,* **17**, 5: 11–31.

Skeet M and Thompson R (1985) Creative nursing: processive care and more? *Journal of Advanced Nursing,* **10**: 15–24.

Skinner B F (1966) An operant analysis of problem solving. In B Kleinmuntz (ed.) (1966) *Problem Solving: Research, Method, and Theory.* New York: John Wiley.

Smith H L (1987) Medical ethics in the primary care setting. *Social Sciences and Medicine,* **25**, 6: 70–9.

Smith R G (1988) *Thinking and Practice in Primary Science Classrooms: A Case Study.* Unpublished PhD Thesis, University of Leeds.

Sparrow S and Pearson A (1985) Teach yourself goal setting. *Nursing Times,* **81**, 42: 24–5.

Staats A W (1966) An integrated-functional learning approach to complex human behaviour. In B Kleinmuntz (ed.) *Problem Solving: Research, Method, and Theory.* New York: John Wiley.

Stewart J (1985) Cognitive science and science education. *European Journal of Science Education,* **7**, 1: 1–17.

Sugden J (1984) The dynamics of change. *Senior Nurse,* **1**, 13: 12–15.

Sullivan E J and Decker P J (1985) *Effective Management in Nursing.* California: Addison-Wesley.

Tanner C A (1986) The nursing care plan as a teaching method: reason or ritual? *Nurse Educator,* **11**, 4: 8–10.

Tanner C A, Padrick K P, Westfall U E and Putzier D J (1987) Diagnostic reasoning strategies of nurses and nursing students. *Nursing Research,* **36**, 6: 358–63.

Tanner C A (1987) Theoretical perspectives for research on clinical judgement. In K J Hannah, M Reimer, W C Mills and S Letourneau (eds) *Clinical Judgement and Decision Making: The Future with Nursing Diagnosis.* Proceedings of the International Conference. May, Calgary, Canada, New York: Wiley.

Teare B R (1980) Recapitulation from the viewpoint of a teacher. In D T Tuma and F Reif (eds) *Problem solving and Education: Issues in Teaching and Research.* New Jersey: Lawrence Erlbaum Associates.

Thompson D R and Sutton T W (1985) Nursing decision making in a coronary care unit. *International Journal of Nursing Studies,* **22**, 3: 259–66.

Thomson R (1959) *The Psychology of Thinking.* Harmondsworth: Penguin.

Tomlinson P (1981) *Understanding Teaching – Interactive Educational Psychology.* London: McGraw-Hill.

Torrington D, Weightman J and Johns K (1985) *Management Methods.* London: Institute of Personnel Management.

Tuckman B W (1978) *Conducting Educational Research,* 2nd edn. New York: Harcourt Brace Jovanovich.

Tuma D T and Reif F (eds) (1980) *Problem Solving and Education: Issues in Teaching and Research.* New Jersey: Lawrence Erlbaum Associates.

UKCC (United Kingdom Central Council for Nursing, Midwifery, and Health Visiting) (1984) *Code of Professional Conduct for the Nurse, Midwife and Health Visitor,* 2nd edn. London: UKCC.

UKCC (United Kingdom Central Council for Nursing, Midwifery, and Health Visiting) (1985) *Project 2000 Facing the Future. Project Paper 6.* London: UKCC.

UKCC (United Kingdom Central Council for Nursing, Midwifery, and Health Visiting) (1987) *Project 2000 the Final Proposals. Project Paper 9.* London: UKCC.

UKCC (United Kingdom Central Council for Nursing, Midwifery, and Health Visiting) (1990) *Discussion Paper on Post-Registration Education and Practice.* London: UKCC.

Vitale B, Lattener N and Nugent P (1978) *A Problem-Solving Approach to Nursing Care Plans.* St Louis: Mosby.

Vu N V (1979) Medical problem-solving assessment: a review of methods and instruments. *Evaluation and the Health Professions,* **2**, 3: 281–307.

Wallas G (1926) The art of thought. In P E Vernon (ed.) (1973), *Creativity: Selective Readings*. Harmondsworth: Penguin.

Walter J B, Pardee G P and Molbo D M (1976) *The Dynamics of Problem Orientated Approaches*. Philadelphia: Lippincott.

Waters K (1986) Cause and effect. *Nursing Times*, **82**, 5: 28–30.

Wenk V A (1981) Analysis and evaluation of the problem-solving process by means of simulated nursing care plans. In S Krampitz and N Pavlovich (eds) *Readings for Nursing Research*. London: Mosby.

Westfall U E, Tanner C A, Putzier D J and Padrick K P (1986) Activating clinical inferences. A component of diagnostic reasoning in nursing. *Research in Nursing and Health*, **9**: 269–77.

Whitis G (1985) Simulation in teaching clinical nursing. *Journal of Nursing Education*, **24**, 4: 161–3.

Whitman N (1983) *Teaching Problem Solving and Creativity in College Courses*. Washington DC: American Association for Higher Education.

Whitmore D A (1985) *Management for Administrators*. London: Heinemann.

Wickelgren W A (1973) *How to Solve Problems: Elements and Theory of Problems and Problem Solving*. San Francisco: W H Freeman.

Wilson H S (1989) *Research in Nursing*, 2nd edn. California: Addison-Wesley.

Woditsch G A (1978) Specifying and achieving competencies. In O Milton (ed.) *On College Teaching: a Guide to Contemporary Practices*. San Francisco: Jossey-Bass.

Wong P, Doyle M and Strauss D (1975) Problem solving through 'process management'. *Journal of Nursing Administration*, **5**: 37–9.

Woodbury P A (1984) Computer-assisted evaluation of problem solving skills of primary health care providers. *The Journal of Continuing Education in Nursing*, **15**, 5: 174–7.

Wooley F, Warnick M, Kane R and Dyer E (1974) *Problem Orientated Nursing*. New York: Springer Publishing Company.

Yeaw E M J (1979) Problem solving as a method of teaching strategies in classroom and clinical teaching. *Journal of Nursing Education*, **18**, 7: 16–22.

Yura H and Walsh M (1978) *The Nursing Process*. New York: Appleton-Century-Crofts.

Appendices

Appendix 1   Vignettes*

Vignette 1   Miss Woods with insomnia

1.1   Sister Smith is a sister on an acute medical ward. She is caring for Miss Woods, a 30-year-old patient, who is under investigation for persistent headache. The patient stops the sister on her morning round and tells her that she is experiencing great difficulty sleeping at night.

1.2   Sister Smith recalls that the staff nurse on night duty had mentioned this in her report. After listening carefully to the patient, the sister checks the night nursing report to confirm that the problem exists. The night report indicates that she has had a restless night.

1.3   She also asks the patient to explain her sleeping pattern before admission to hospital. This line of enquiry reveals that the patient is sleeping badly in comparison to her sleeping habits at home. The sister notes the following factors which might be keeping her awake:

a. noisy ward;
b. unusual environment;
c. her analgesic medication.

Having agreed the list with the patient, she places the probable causes into an order of priority.

1.4   Following discussion with Miss Woods and her physician, the sister sets two goals:

a. to ensure the patient is pain-free;
b. to ensure that the patient is nursed in an environment conducive to sleep.

1.5   Later the same day, the following changes are made to Miss Woods' care:

a. the patient's medication is reviewed; a different analgesic is prescribed (the physician does not wish to prescribe a hypnotic at this stage);
b. Miss Woods' bed is placed in a side-room to ensure maximum quietness at night.

1.6   Sister Smith asks both the patient and the night staff how well she is sleeping as a result of these changes. There is a slight improvement but the sister feels further action is necessary.

1.7   She asks Miss Woods if there is anything else that could be keeping her awake. She suggests to the patient that it could possibly be an aspect of her

* The original vignettes in each case were no more than a single page.

occupation. The patient indicates that there are no problems with her work or financial/domestic affairs.

1.8   The patient's remaining stay in hospital is uneventful with still further improvement in her sleeping. As a result, she is much happier and no further action seems necessary.

Vignette 2   Mr Franks, a patient who has had a partial gastrectomy

2.1   Mr Franks is 40 years old and had a partial gastrectomy for a chronic peptic ulcer three days ago. Student Nurse Jones notices that the patient's wound is inflamed when changing his dressing. She covers the wound with a gauze swab and reports her worries to Sister Potts.

2.2   Sister Potts sets several goals in terms of this patient's care:

a. to ensure that the patient remains comfortable in terms of his wound and general well-being;
b. to improve the patient's nutritional state and encourage wound healing;
c. to protect the other patients and staff from his possible wound infection.

2.3   Between the third and sixth post-operative days Mr Franks receives the following specific care, in addition to his general nursing care:

a. the patient's surgeon orders 'A wound swab for microscopy, culture and sensitivity' before prescribing a seven-day course of parenteral antibiotics;
b. the patient and his wife are given simple explanations of the change in his care and progress. They receive an initial reassurance that the inflammation will subside once the antibiotics are being received;
c. the patient's level of discomfort is checked periodically and analgesic medication given as appropriate;
d. one team is allocated to care for him until the result of the wound swab is known to minimise cross-infection;
e. the patient is soon able to tolerate oral fluids; he is then given a high-protein diet to encourage wound healing;
f. mouth care is continued to improve the patient's comfort and minimise the risk of respiratory tract infection;
g. his vital signs are recorded four-hourly, particularly his temperature;
h. the wound is re-dressed daily by the same nurse and is always the last wound to be re-dressed.

2.4   Daily written and verbal reports are made about Mr Franks, in particular the progress of his wound. Fortunately, his wound settles down and heals without any further problem. The sister also notes that his wound swab proves negative and the very slight rise in his body temperature has now subsided. Mr Franks quickly becomes mobile and soon enjoys a light nutritious diet. The health-care team fully expect him to make a good recovery.

Vignette 3   The parents who complain about their child's care

3.1   Mr and Mrs Brown are the parents of Jane, an eight-month-old girl, admitted to the paediatric ward with an acute respiratory tract infection. Neither of the parents is able to stay with Jane for very long since Mr Brown is a senior business executive who works away, and his wife cares for her elderly, infirm mother at home.

3.2 Sister Budd is told by Student Nurse Smith that the parents of Jane have complained about the nursing care their daughter is receiving. Student Nurse Smith is upset by the attitude of the parents, who shouted at her claiming that the nappy was 'soaking wet and smelly' and 'could not have been changed in the past eight hours'. Sister Brown does down to speak with Mr and Mrs Brown, who repeat the allegation.

3.3 Sister Budd immediately takes the following steps. She apologises to the parents and reassures them that this occurrence will definitely not happen again. She goes on to explain that the ward is very busy at the moment.

3.4 The sister and Nurse Smith prepare to wash Jane and put on a clean nappy. Throughout the procedure Nurse Smith 'talks' to Jane while Sister Budd chats to Mr and Mrs Brown about their daughter.

3.5 Student Nurse Smith stays with the family and completes the child's bed charts, while Sister Budd makes adjustments to Jane's care plan and writes a full report about the incident in the nursing records. The nurses coming on to the next shift are given an explanation about the event and asked to note how things go.

3.6 After talking with Mr and Mrs Brown, Sister Budd feels that they seem much happier. She is further reassured on the next day when she is greeted very pleasantly by Mr and Mrs Brown. Similarly, she notes that the parents are chatting happily with Student Nurse Smith, who is attending to Jane. There is a slight improvement in Jane's condition.

3.7 Jane Brown makes an excellent recovery over the next few days and is soon breathing, eating and drinking normally. It is expected that the child will be home within the next three days.

Vignette 4 A young man with traumatic enucleation of his left eye

4.1 John Smith is a 19-year-old patient whose left eye was enucleated following a motor-cycle accident three weeks ago. The socket has now healed and he is almost ready for discharge from hospital to home. Apart from the physical injury, the accident has affected John in other ways: his mother tells Sister Daws, who has just returned from a two-week holiday, that her son 'has changed' and that 'he appears withdrawn'. Sister Daws suspects that John's quietness is abnormal.

4.2 Sister Daws spends some time with John asking him about aspects of his injury and recovery. She talks with him about his outlook on life, his occupation and interests, etc.

4.3 The sister summarises John's nursing problems as:

a. clinical: preparation of his socket for the prosthesis;
b. psychological: helping him to accept his injury and to teach him to care for his socket.

4.4 The sister believes that mastery of his eye care is paramount, since this will help him to speed up his rehabilitation, in particular helping to solve his psychological problems.

4.5 After attempting further discussions with John, the sister sets the following goals in terms of his rehabilitation:

a. to improve John's outlook on life;
b. to assist him to become independent in the care of his socket;
c. to ensure continuation of his care by involving his family and other agencies, particularly after discharge from hospital.

4.6 Over the next two days, John receives the following specific care, over and above his general nursing care:

a. Sister Daws explains to John that with the support of his family there is no reason why he should not return to a normal lifestyle;
b. she stresses the fact that since there is no damage to the skin surrounding his socket, the cosmetic appearance should be of high quality, once the prosthesis is in place;
c. the follow-up appointment system is explained to John;
d. the patient is shown how to care for his socket in preparation for the fitting of his prosthesis;
e. finally, John is introduced to an ex-patient who has had an excellent prosthesis fitted.

4.7 Four days later John is discharged home to the care of the district nurse.

Vignette 5   Mrs Forest with ischaemic heart disease

5.1 Mrs Forest is a 59-year-old lady admitted to a medical ward with ischaemic heart disease. She is asymptomatic apart from angina pectoris on exertion, a condition which is getting worse. The main reason for admitting Mrs Forest is to improve her prognosis by changing her lifestyle.

5.2 During the admission process the patient tells Sister Smith that both her brother and father died following heart attacks before they reached the age of 60 years. Sister Smith decides to sit down and talk with the patient to get a fuller picture about her job, family and lifestyle. She notes that Mrs Forest, although happily married, admits to 'being a worrier', principally about her family and her job as factory worker. She also records that the patient smokes 30 cigarettes a day and is 25 kg overweight.

5.3 Sister Smith then discusses Mrs Forest's case with the physician dietician and the ward team of nurses. As a result, the following goals are set with the patient's agreement:

a. to reduce Mrs Forest's anxiety regarding her prognosis;
b. to reduce her smoking with a view to stopping altogether;
c. to assist her to lose weight, using the diet recommended by the dietician;
d. to educate her to lead a healthier lifestyle;
e. to involve her family in her care.

5.4 Ten days later Sister Smith checks Mrs Forest's records which show that she has lost 4 kg in weight, but the efforts to reduce her smoking have been less successful. Mrs Forest is smoking 20 cigarettes instead of her usual 30.

5.5 The patient is confident that she will be able to stop smoking and realises the need to eat a healthier diet. Her family agree to support her in this respect.

5.6   Shortly after, she is discharged home under the care of her general practictioner with monthly out-patient department appointments to see her consultant. Mrs Forest is also referred to the liaison health visitor (for coronary patients) who will co-ordinate her follow-up care.

Vignette 6   Mr Shaw, a patient with a circulatory problem

6.1   Sister Briggs is checking all the patients who have had surgery today. When she goes to Mr Shaw she sees that he has taken his arm out of his elevation sling and is hanging it out of bed. The patient returned from the recovery room three hours ago following surgery for a repair of a tendon in his left wrist. Although sleepy, Mr Shaw has been talking to the patient in the next bed.

6.2   The sister examines the patient's arm more closely and questions him about it. She notes the patient's fingers are swollen, blue and cold. Mr Shaw says that his fingers are 'tingling' and his arm is painful.

6.3   The sister immediately cuts the Velband (a bandage-type dressing) on his left arm but leaves the back-slab in place supported by a loose crepe bandage. She then informs the surgeon, who asks to be kept informed.

6.4   The sister also sets several short-term goals for this patient:

a. to observe the patient's fingers and inform the surgeon of any further problems;
b. to educate the patient on the importance of keeping his arm elevated to reduce swelling;
c. to ensure the patient is pain-free.

6.5   The patient receives the following specific nursing care:

a. his arm is elevated in the sling and he is reminded of the importance of keeping it in place;
b. the nurse caring for him is asked to check that the patient is keeping his arm in the elevated position;
c. the patient is given analgesic medication as prescribed.

6.6   Within a few days he is discharged home with the expectation that he will return to his job as a bank clerk.

Vignette 7   Mr Jones, an insulin-dependent diabetic

7.1   Mr Jones is a newly diagnosed insulin-dependent diabetic. He has responded well to treatment and is controlled on twice-daily insulin and a restricted carbohydrate diet. Sister Brown begins to teach the patient to administer his own insulin, but discovers that he is reluctant to do this. Consequently, he is not making progress towards independence in his self-care.

7.2   The sister decides to get to the bottom of this problem. She notes that the patient is a 45-year-old school teacher, happily married with teenage children. She sits down and talks with him about his condition. Mr Jones explains that neither he nor any member of his family have suffered from serious illness and that they feel 'bowled over' by the sudden onset of this crisis. He goes on to explain that he has lost all confidence in himself and feels inadequate.

7.3   Sister Brown takes the following action:

a. she reassures the patient that this is a normal reaction to his present illness;
b. she asks the liaison health visitor for diabetic patients to spend some time with Mrs Jones and his family to reinforce the patient's education programme;
c. she asks the dietician to talk with him and his wife regarding his future diet;
d. she informs the patient's physician of these difficulties.

7.4   At a case conference 14 days later, involving Sister Brown, the health visitor, dietician and physician, it is recorded that Mr Jones is almost proficient in his own care and feels much happier as a result. All concerned now believe he is ready for discharge home. The health visitor has already agreed to continue his care at home and generally monitor his progress. The physician will also see him in the out-patient department in a few weeks.

Appendix 2   Instruction Sheet given to each Informant prior to Interview

Introduction

Thank you for agreeing to take part in this interview, it should take between 30 and 60 minutes to complete.

I am interested in the way nurses solve nursing problems. From my preliminary investigations it has become clear that there is some confusion about what nurses consider nursing problem-solving to be. The information you give during this interview will help to unravel some of the mystery which surrounds this important nursing skill.

What I have done is to collect five different, but real nursing incidents from various wards. As you read the vignettes (a short description of an incident) you will quickly form an impression of each one.

What I would like you to do is to sort them into rank-order from best to worst, using a scale of 1 to 5 (1 = best, 5 = worst). If any of the vignettes are worthy of equal rank then feel free to rate them as such.

Once you have ranked the vignettes, please talk yourself through each one and tell me:

1. what you like or dislike about each one;
2. what is missing or should be omitted from each one;
3. what makes one the same as or different from another.

Please refer to the number at the beginning of each paragraph if you wish to make a specific point.

If you wish to make notes whilst you work through each vignette then please do so.

May I emphasise that this is *not* a test of your clinical knowledge, but I would like you to take into consideration all aspects of the vignette, not just the medical treatment and nursing care. Feel free to ask questions before you begin working.

I shall be recording this conversation on my tape recorder to help me carry out a better analysis later on. However, I would like to reassure you that the data you provide will be anonymous and kept confidential.

Appendix 3 Guide for Analysing Informants' Perceptions of Vignettes

1. *Problem identification* (pi)
   1.1 Comments on the way the problem has or should have been identified.
   1.2 Comments on the way the problem has or should have been confirmed.
   1.3 Comments on the way the sub-problem/s have or should have been distinguished from the main problem.

2. *Problem assessment* (a)
   2.1 Comments on the way the problem has or should have been explored to determine the extent of the problem.
   2.2 Comments on the way appropriate information has or should have been gathered.
   2.3 Comments on the way problems/sub-problems have or should have been sorted/classified.

*3. *Planning interventions* (p)
   3.1 Comments on the way goals have or should have been set.
   3.2 Comments on the way goals have or should have been prioritised.
   3.3 Comments on the way strategies for achieving the goals have or should have been made.

4. *Implementation* (i)
   4.1 Comments on the way nursing plans* have or should have been carried out.
   4.2 Comments on the actual nursing interventions irrespective of whether a particular goal (or goals) has (or have) been recognised.

5. *Evaluation* (e)
   5.1 Comments on the way evidence has or should have been collected and appraised for the purpose of deciding on the success of the nursing plan.*
   5.2 Comments on the way a decision has or should have been made about whether a successful solution has been achieved.

* For the purposes of this research, the nursing plan is the goal plus the planned intervention.

5.3   Comments on the way a decision has or should have been made to recommence the cycle.

5.4   Comments on the phase at which the process has or should have been re-entered, following evaluation.

6.   *Not definable* (nd)

6.1   Statement which cannot be matched to one of the above.

Appendix 4   Transcript of an Interview with a Third-year Learner Nurse

Key: I = informant
 R = researcher
Italics represents the informant's emphasis.

R: Thank you for agreeing to be interviewed. I am interested in the way nurses solve clinical problems. I am interviewing over 100 nurses on this subject and as your lecturer has told you, five nurses are from this school of nursing and you are one of the five who were kind enough to volunteer. This research is for my higher degree and I would like to stress that I am working independently of your school. You are, therefore, under no obligation to participate. However, I would like to reassure you that everything said here will be in strict confidence. I can guarantee anonymity.

I: It's quite all right. It sounded interesting, that's why I volunteered. What do I have to do?

R: I have an information and instruction sheet here, which I would like you to read. If you are happy to continue after you have read it, we will take it from there.

I: [Reads introductory sheet] That's OK.

R: Just to reiterate. Some time ago I interviewed five experienced ward sisters. I asked each one to describe a problem which happened to her recently and how she dealt with it. I am now going to show you the written accounts of these five problem-solving situations. What I want you to do is to read all five and then place them in order from best to worst, in terms of the way the problems were solved. Then I would like you to talk me through each one and tell me what you liked and disliked about each vignette. Please take your time. Feel free to make notes as you go along. Do you have any questions before you start?

I: No, that seems clear. [Reads the vignettes]. I like number three the best, followed by number four. With the rest, there isn't much to choose between them, I rate them all third.

R: That's fine, thank you. Can you now talk me through them and tell me what you feel about each one in more detail. Can you begin by telling me which one you are talking about please. It's all yours.

I: Number one [pause]. It is pretty good that she, in fact, checks the night report and asks the night staff how she is getting on. And the next important thing is that she asks her to explain her sleeping pattern because she doesn't know if she sleeps badly at home and it is *important* to know how she sleeps at home [pause].

R: Can I just go back a bit before you move on because you said that it is good that she checks the night nursing report. Why is that?

I: Because some people think it suspicious that she doesn't believe the patient. I think she gets all the information.

R: Yes, I thought that is what you meant, but I thought I would clarify. Fine, thank you.

I: I think she identified the factors quite well, noisy ward and unusual environment; that could be affecting her sleeping [pause].

R: I see.

I: I think she has got the goals right as well, in that the patient was pain-free, first of all [pause]. It's difficult in hospital to have an environment conducive to sleep. So, I think she handled it in the best way she possibly can by using a side-ward if Mrs Woods prefers it [pause]. I think it would be quieter at night. And giving analgesics as she requires it. And then she evaluates as well, by asking if there is a result, you know, in the changes she has made. And both staff and the patient feel there is [pause]. She also asks if there are psychological sort of problems, or social problems. The patient says there isn't. So this probably hasn't got anything to do with the fact that she isn't sleeping well. It could just be the environment.

R: Fine.

I: And it was quite successful [pause]. She had an improvement. Although she wasn't sleeping really, really well, when she went home [pause]. That's all.

R: Thank you. Would you like to refresh your memory about the next one before you start to speak?

I: [Re-reads Vignette 2]. Number two [pause]. It seems that Sister Potts is *actually* setting the goals, in terms of the patient's care without *actually* going to see him and talking about it. To see what his problems *actually* are [pause].

R: I see.

I: His problem might not be stated as she would state them [pause]. He would probably state them totally differently in fact [pause]. I think, however, that the care she decides to give in the end is quite good. The fact that the wound swab is taken before antibiotics are given, obviously, and she explains why these things are happening to him and his wife [pause]. I presume there is good communication between him and his wife, because he wants his wife to know all about it. I don't know. I presume so [pause]. They check that he is comfortable, and so on [pause]. There is perhaps one thing that I thought of. One team was allocated to care for him, which I think is quite a good idea [pause].

R: Yes.

I: But, I mean, the *most* important thing about giving care is that he gets on, I suppose, with the nursing staff and they like him [pause].

R: Yes.

I: And as I say, it was quite successful. She didn't *actually* discuss with him what he thought his care should be, or what he felt about it. That's about it [pause].

R: Fine and the next one. All yours.

I: [Re-reads Vignette 3]. Number three [pause]. It's unfortunate that the parents are unable to stay with Jane for very long. Perhaps they feel guilty about this, I don't know, perhaps that is what upset them. Or perhaps Mrs Brown is worried about her mother at home. That *could* be upsetting her as well, because, perhaps she has had a difficult day with her [pause]. I understand why the student nurse got upset, but it would be important for the student nurse to realise *why* the parents are feeling like this.

R: Yes. OK.

I: And perhaps they are exaggerating about saying the past eight hours. I think Sister Budd should have [pause] reassured herself that this wasn't true, or, you know, checked that it had been changed recently.

R: Yes, fine.

I: I agree that she should have apologised to the parents. But she reassures them that this occurrence will not happen again. She doesn't know if it occurred the *first* time. It might have been changed recently [pause]. And it's not a very good excuse really to explain that the ward is very busy. The parents probably don't care *particularly* about that. They just want the *best* care for their daughter, I suppose. Even though that may be true [pause].

R: Yes, OK.

I: I think it is an *excellent* idea to actually have the parents there while the nurses are caring for Jane. Although, I would, I think, prefer the parents to do it for themselves, if they could, while they were there [pause]. *But*, it seems to have reassured the parents that their daughter is getting decent care, because they are quite happy about it and they seem much more cheerful [pause] and they are much more pleasant to the nursing staff afterwards. And so, it was handled reasonably well, but I would have said that [pause] the parents should, you know, get more involved in the care, whilst they are there. It is always encouraged, I think, on the wards here and it is a good idea, because they have to be away from them while they are at home [pause].

R: Yes.

I: So, I think it was handled pretty well as I say, [pause] but I don't think the sister handled it as well as she could have done [pause].

R: Yes, I would agree with you. Thank you and the next.

I: [Re-reads Vignette 4]. Number four. This is a very difficult problem really [pause]. Psychological problems I think are probably *more* important, or affecting more than his actual physical problems despite the fact that the sister thinks differently. She thinks that it is paramount, his mastery of the eye care is the *most* important thing. It *is* important to be able to care for his own physical problems [pause]. And it will help him psychologically, but helping him to accept his injury is probably going to take a *much, much* longer time than that. And if she hasn't been given enough of, sort of, training in psychological care, or also she might not be treating John correctly at all saying the correct things to him. And I believe that someone with more experience in psychological care could have been included in his treatment programme to help him over his problems [pause]. I should have mentioned this in the beginning, but I think that it was good that she [pause] actually realised that he was behaving differently from normal and his mother would have probably mentioned it if that wasn't the case.

R: Yes, good.
I: But she probably has a bit of experience in dealing with these patients before and realises he has psychological problems [pause]. The goals are pretty good: actually it says to improve John's 'outlook on life'. Perhaps she didn't ought to phrase it like that [pause]. It's probably not his outlook that is the problem at all, actually. He is probably not depressed yet. It is just that, you know, he doesn't quite know how to deal with the massive problems presented to him [pause].
R: I see, how would you rewrite that?
I: I thought you would ask me that [laughs]. Well, I would try to find out what his specific problem was. Whether it was [pause]. How it was going to look, or whether he felt he couldn't physically deal with it, or how he felt it would affect, say, his marriage or relationships with a female or something like that. I would try to find out, you know, what the specific problem was. If there particularly was one [pause].
R: I see, thank you.
I: And she reassures him that there is no problem with his lifestyle. As I say, that was quite good [pause]. Reassures him about the cosmetic appearance of it [pause]. And the last points are very good. I think it is important that he sees someone who has had a successful operation like this. That's a very good idea [pause].
R: OK.
I: 'Four days later he is discharged home to the care of the district nurse', it says [pause]. Four days later is not an awful long time. His psychological care, I think, will take a lot longer than four days. He should be followed up from that point of view as well, to see how he was coping.
R: When you say followed up, in what sense?
I: I didn't quite. The psychological care given in hospital by the nurses doesn't seem to be followed up particularly at home, unless you have got someone who specialises, for example, the stoma-care nurse, or someone like that. She helps with psychological problems. The district nurse probably couldn't. And I think that someone, who has more expertise in this area should have seen him afterwards, yeah; this kind of thing [pause].
R: Yes. OK.
I: He probably just wants someone to talk to, in fact. Reassure him that everything was OK. The district nurse wouldn't have time to do that either; very busy. So, I think someone else should do that particular care. OK.
R: Great, thank you. The next one.
I: [Re-reads Vignette 5]. Number five. This lady is probably very, very anxious about having this problem anyway. Especially with her family history of her brother and father dying of heart attacks. I think the idea that Sister Smith decides to sit down and talk to her about her lifestyle is really good [pause]. So that she can note the problems [pause].
R: Yes. OK.
I: She admits to being a worrier and sometimes the personality type can be a problem with coronary heart disease. This Type A personality, there is not a lot you can do about it. Apart from helping her to cope with stress [pause]. *Perhaps* she copes with stress by smoking thirty a day and overeating as well, which is why she is overweight [pause]. I think it is very good that she includes other people in her care. The dietician, who has got expertise, well sort of, making sure that she sort of loses

some weight really. And the goals are set with the patient's agreement as well [pause]. I think first of all really, understanding the problem, and her lifestyle should have been assessed, really. But, fortunately, it says later on she is confident and that she will be able to stop smoking and realises the need to eat a healthier diet. But, I think that when she goes home, will she be able to keep it up? I mean in hospital things are done for her, really. The dietician gives the diet. I mean, does Mrs Forest realise the salt content and fat content of certain foods? I think really, what *she* eats, basically, at home, if she, sort of, has to fry different things for her family. If her husband has a manual job, or whatever, it should be taken into account [pause]. I think, because things are, sort of, arranged for her in hospital, you can't really check up on her when she goes home. Fortunately, she has got a health visitor seeing her at home, and they might be able to sort that out. But I think that [pause], before she leaves really, this sort of thing needs to be discussed with her. The health education programme in hospital isn't *always* very successful. It could be better done outside. I don't think enough has been done from that point of view [pause].

R: Great, anything else with that one.

I: I don't think there is anything I need to say. I'm sure there is a lot more in that!

R: No, you have brought out a lot of the points I would have liked you to raise. You said some things earlier that I would like to explore further. Probably the best way for me to do that is to show you another vignette. Would you please read this one and comment on it in the way you have been doing.

I: [Reads Vignette 7]. Vignette number seven. It is obviously important that the patient is taught the correct way to administer his own insulin and I can understand that he is going to be reluctant to do this [pause].

R: Yes, fine.

I: The needles now are pretty good. They are really tiny, and so on. So perhaps, if all of these things are pointed out to him; how deep it goes; the fact that it is not particularly painful. It is more like a pin prick than an injection. Perhaps he is frightened of needles, I don't know [pause].

R: Fine.

I: It is *very, very important* though that he has independence in this, because he has got to do it all the time at home if he is on it twice daily. It is good that the sister involves the whole family and notes his social background [pause]. It is a serious illness really, because it can have a lot of problems if it is not controlled. However, if it is controlled *well*, he shouldn't have too many problems. This should, really, be explained to him. It is only if your levels of sugar and so on get really bad that you are going to get the real problems. He is a bit old to be on insulin twice-daily, perhaps, I don't know. I have had only experience with, sort of, younger people. Usually at forty-five years of age they are on hypo-glycaemic agents and diet. But insulin? [pause].

R: He came into hospital with hyperglycaemic coma. That would denote quite serious diabetes. It doesn't say that and you weren't to know that. But that is what happened to him.

I: Yes, I see. OK. I am glad she reassures him that it is a normal reaction to his illness, because, I think it is. Loss of confidence and suddenly he sort of has this catastrophe. Again, she should explain that if it is monitored properly he should have less problems. So, perhaps he would be more keen to come to the appointments, and that. If she should explain that to him [pause]. The health visitor can see him outside of hospital, so it is a good idea to involve her and the dietician as well. And I think one of the *most* important things for diabetics is the British Diabetic Association, which is absolutely excellent. It, sort of, helps you realise that you are not isolated in your own particular problem and lots of people suffer with it. And it, sort of, helps all age groups; not just the young ones with things. I know more about the holidays and so on that they can go on. I don't know much about the older patients. But they do things for them as well [pause]. And it just helps, really. I like the problem pages as well. Reading through that makes you realise that you are not the only one with problems. Perhaps you could get advice on how to solve your own there. So, I think that should be mentioned, and that is very important [pause].

R: Yes, good points.

I: But, it is not particularly handled brilliantly, but it is *not bad*. I don't see what else I could do from the sister's point of view [pause]. And as I say, his condition is OK after this anyway, so perhaps it is not such a bad thing as he thought. But as I say, some of the points I have mentioned, she should have mentioned anyway, which I think should help a lot. That's about it.

R: Right, thank you very much. This has been a valuable interview. I have gathered much useful information here. Unfortunately, I am unable to give you feedback, because I may want to come back and talk to you again. The best I can say at the moment is that I do hope to produce some kind of report which will, hopefully, appear in print later. Once again, thank you very much for giving your time. Can I just ask you for one more thing. Please do not discuss the interview with any of your colleagues, because I may be interviewing them later.

Appendix 5   A Coded Transcript of an Interview with a Nurse Teacher

Key: I   = informant
    pi = problem identification
    a   = problem assessment
    p   = planning interventions
    i   = implementation
    e   = evaluation
    nd = not definable

The researcher's comments have been deliberately omitted from this transcript.

Vignette 1

I/pi: It has been identified that she is suffering from sleepless nights. This has been highlighted by the night nurses.

a: Sister has obviously been talking to the patient and has some more information about her problems. I would like to have known more. She is talking about the noisy ward, unusual environment, the bed, her analgesic medication. It is a thirty-year old, who is under investigation for persistent headache. I would have liked to have seen more information on the psychological aspects here. I think there are assumptions that her sleeping pattern has changed while she is in hospital, because of the change in the environment, more than anything else. Maybe at night the patient has this headache and asks herself, 'Have I got something nasty like a tumour?' I think it is very much taken that it must be the ward environment, rather than more of looking into detail at the psychological aspects and how the patient is feeling.

p: I would suggest that the goals set are very limited. [Reads 1.4a]. Can we as nurses guarantee that? The answer is no. You might be able to relieve some of the pain; dull the feeling of pain. To make the patient pain-free is not an achievable goal. [Reads 1.4b]. Well yes, it may be achievable to a certain extent. I think one should be looking further afield and saying well, if the patient wants to sit in the day room; sit in the chair during the night, are we allowing those facilities, or are we saying that if we are putting you in a side ward you will be all right? To actually state 'putting them in a side room' actually ensures maximum quietness at night is another assumption. Whether you are out on the main ward, or in a side ward with the door closed, you are still going to hear noises.

i/a: Maybe somebody talking to the patient at night when she is having the sleepless nights. Actually sitting and allowing her to talk freely about how she is feeling. Are there any particular worries? Is she worried about her condition? Is she worried about her job or finances? That is not mentioned.

p: It is just decided that if you change the patient's medication and if you put her in a side room, then that will improve the situation.

e/pi: In fact it hasn't, because it is stated here that there is only slight improvement. But no further action needs to be taken. Nothing is referred to regarding further action. No identification of further problems is made there.

a: She asks Miss Woods if there is anything else that could be keeping her awake. The sister suggests at that point that she [reads 1.7]. That again, is an assumption.

e: I mean, to end it by saying that the patient's stay is uneventful [reads 1.8]. That doesn't follow the pattern at all. That may be how the nurses perceive it. I would say that the patient wouldn't perceive it that way. I imagine that during the patient's remaining stay in hospital, she had very little sleep and is probably greatly relieved to be going home to make up for lost sleep.

nd: I don't think sister has handled it at all well. I think there are too many assumptions and not enough involvement of, or with, the patient.

e/a: Certainly, at times, when she is not able to sleep. Someone should be trying to find out exactly why. It is very poor indeed.

Vignette 2

I/nd: I think that the way the problem was solved was very well done.

p: The sister has identified the goals in terms of the patient's needs. Not only about the comfort of the patient but also the nutrition of the patient and the wound healing. Also protection of the other staff.

i: Secondly, both the patient and wife were involved in his care. They were both kept well informed as to what was happening to him. The fact that in order to prevent the cross-infection they allocated one nurse, rather than a different nurse, was good.

e: There was a complete follow-through as to whether the wound was improving or not.

i: They also related to both him and his wife.

a: They looked at other aspects relating to his wound: comfort and not just thinking of him in terms of the wound; as a whole person really.

e: And the fact that it was documented well. Both written and verbal reports were being made to assess [sic] his progress.

nd: I don't think there is anything lacking here. In fact, the sister has solved the problem really well.

a: I would have followed roughly what has been stated here. I presume,
        that after the wound was reported to the sister, the sister went to have
        a look at the wound.
a/i: Maybe, there should have been some action to alleviate his anxiety at
        the time the sister went to see the wound. He might think, 'Oh, here is
        sister coming to look at my wound.' There might have been some
        concern expressed at that time. The sister might need to explain to the
        patient that this is a normal thing to happen after an operation.
nd: Then I would have followed what has been highlighted here.
i/p/a: If you look at the priorities set down here. I mean [reads 2.3b], that is
        quite high up in the second part. In fact, the priority should be to give
        Mr Franks explanations and it would need to be in the goals as well,
        which she would have done if she had gone to look at the wound.

Vignette 3

l/pi: It appears that the parents are not happy with the nursing care being
        given to their daughter. This has been reported to the sister by the
        learner. It is quite good that the learner reported it. The learner is upset
        by the attitude of the parents. [Reads last sentence of 3.2]. From then
        on it goes a little haywire to say the least.
a: I think, firstly, the sister should have been discussing more with the
        parents the reason why they are making this allegation. I would
        suggest that because they are unable to stay with their daughter, as
        much that he is away from home and has probably got pressures of
        work. The wife is caring [reads last line of 3.1]. It makes it difficult for
        either one of them to be with their daughter and she is only eight
        months old. I would imagine they are projecting their anger onto other
        people. They are angry with themselves, because they are not able to
        stay with their daughter. So I think anger is being projected by saying
        the nursing care is not very good.
i: I think the sister ought to have talked to the learner anyway, because,
        obviously, by their attitude. The learner probably doesn't realise that
        they are projecting anger onto her and everyone else, because they
        feel that they are unable to meet their daughter's needs.
a/i: Probably they are anxious because they are not there all the time and
        don't know if she is improving or not. If they are coming sort of one-
        off a day. If they are just coming in every day, or every two days, they
        aren't going to be aware of the progress their child is making, unless
        one of the staff speaks to them, saying she is much better today.
i: The fact that the sister apologises to the parents is admitting that the
        nursing care wasn't good. I think, again, that is wrong.
pi/a: Because she has not actually identified why the parents are saying
        these things, that the nursing care is not up to their expectations.
i: She sort of reassures them that this will not happen again. So, she is
        admitting that, yes, we haven't been giving the correct nursing care
        and we will not let it happen again, which I think is totally wrong. I think
        that the next part, where the sister and the learner go to the daughter,
        is a good thing. But maybe, because it is only a learner looking after
        their daughter, is she capable of giving the correct nursing care? Does
        she know what she is doing? If a senior member of staff was there,

then the parents' anxiety levels would be relieved, because they would think someone is observing her; there is somebody talking to us. I think the fact that the learner was going in to carry out a task, rather than involving the parents and keeping them up-to-date with how Jane was progressing, was wrong.

i/e: It does seem, with the fact that the sister does go in with the learner to look after Jane, that it does help the situation, because the parents are happier and appear happier the next time they come in.

a: I think, in general, what it does show is a lack of communication between the nursing staff. And the parents lack of understanding; what the parents must be feeling; the pressures; the stress. The fact that they have an eight-month-old girl in hospital and they are not able to visit.

p: No reference has been made to overcoming that. Possibly, a social worker should have been brought in to, maybe, give some support to the wife, regards her elderly mother at home, so she could have had some support there and be allowed to come and see Jane. As far as Mr Brown is concerned, he probably would have difficulty with the senior post he has got. But I think something should have been done to relieve the burden on the wife. That could easily have been arranged. That is missing from this.

a: So, I think it is a lack of communication; a lack of understanding of the problem, with regard to how the parents are feeling.

nd: The sister needs guidance in the management of these problems when they arise.

a/i: I think she needs to realise that there is an awful lot more to identify and discuss what the causes are relating to this problem before jumping in and saying yes, I take responsibility. So, she is not really aware of her own responsibility and accountability.

i: I don't think she is aware, by saying that in fact, the parents could easily put a complaint into the health authority saying that 'we are complaining about the care our child is being given'. All right, she has documented it, but one hopes that, maybe, her senior manager would actually sit down with her and say, 'Look, you didn't handle that particularly well.' She doesn't seem to be aware that she is taking full responsibility for the incident and if the parents complain, they are likely to win the case, because she hasn't got a leg to stand on really, because she has admitted to it. She has documented what she has done, so it is all there.

nd: I think, what she should have done was to consult somebody earlier on if she felt unable to cope with the situation herself.

Vignette 4

l/pi: It is all about a nineteen-year-old who lost an eye in a motor-cycle accident. He is almost ready for discharge. It appears that nobody has picked up the problems John is experiencing. The fact that he is withdrawn and his mother has picked it up and tells sister.

a: [Reads 4.2, 4.3a, 4.3b]. I think they are the wrong way round. I would suggest psychological. He is only nineteen, the start of enjoying his life as an adult. I would suggest psychological would be the main problem affecting John more than the prosthesis. I think that is a secondary problem [4.3a]. She has written down the problems as (a) clinical, and (b) psychological, which is wrong. Psychological should be the first one. [Reads 4.4]. Which, I think, is totally wrong. The thing that she has missed is the fact that he has had an enucleation of his eye. That he is aware of it and that he will be looked at and stared at by other people, who will notice he has got a different eye. There is a change in his body image. He is only nineteen, probably enjoying life; socialising with girlfriends. This is all going to be upset, because of his accident.

p: To actually say that putting in his prosthesis will overcome all these problems is ridiculous. It totally shows a lack of empathy on the part of a senior person to a patient. It seems to be a task-oriented idea, you know. If he masters putting the prosthesis in his left eye, he will be all right. That's all he has got to do. So I think that setting up the goals in terms of his rehabilitation are totally out of context. I mean, [reads 4.5a] one could argue if that is an achievable goal and how are you going to do it. If you are going to do it like that, it is sort of step-by-step goal and identifying probably what could be achieved. But to put that I don't think is achievable. All right [reads 4.5b], again, she needs to mention how she will do it. It may be necessary to do it in stages. Allowing him to handle the prosthesis before thinking how to put it in himself. So that would have to be done in steps as well. [Reads 4.5c]. To a certain extent, yes, but that is very broad and not specific enough. One could argue that his family are concerned. His mother is the one who observed the changes in his personality. Really, what do you mean by other agencies? Again, it is not specific enough. You could think in terms of someone who has had a similar traumatic experience, who could come in and talk to John about his own experiences and leading a normal lifestyle afterwards. The goals which have been set are not really achievable. They are too broad and need to be identified in steps, rather than a broad content.

i: Assumptions are being made. Just explaining to him that with the support of his family [reads 4.6a], which again doesn't follow. The sister is missing the point; the fact that he is only nineteen. All right, he will have family support, but, maybe, when he may not want to face people who he stays with at home. But, really, what she is saying is, 'Don't worry John, with the support of your family, everything will be all right. You will be leading a normal lifestyle, nothing has happened.'

a: There is a total misunderstanding of the factor of his age. What has actually happened to him is a traumatic experience for anybody. Particularly for anyone of that age group.

i: It tends to be very much getting the prosthesis fitted. Making sure it is a good fit. Nothing about the psychological aspects.

a: She has summarised nursing problems as clinical, first and foremost.

p: It then follows that all the other aspects which follow have been identified regarding the setting of goals; specific care.

i: It really relates to overcoming the problem in its clinical aspects, rather than psychological aspects.

pi: I mean, you have to question that it is the mother who observes the change and reports the problem to the ward sister and not the nursing staff who spot the problem.

a: I mean, it says that John's quietness is abnormal. There is nothing relating to why and what is behind it. OK she spends time with John talking about aspects of his injury, but at that time, if he is withdrawn, he is not going to give too much away. He is not going to give her too much information to work on. I would suggest that if you are going to do that it would take a lot of interviews with the patient. As far as the patient is concerned, what he really does feel.

p: Then allowing him to set his own goals to see what he can achieve, rather than the nurses setting the goals.

Vignette 5

l/pi/a: I think it was tackled quite well from the point of view that she was very anxious on admission and sister obviously picked this up and spent some time with her getting information about her job, family and lifestyle. So, identifying from that the reasons why she has got ischaemic heart disease. Obviously there is a need to look at health education aspects.

p: I would suggest that with discussing the case with the physician, dietician and ward team of nurses is fine, but, maybe, somewhere amongst the goals set there, the patient should have been involved, in setting her own goals, or what she feels she could achieve during her stay in hospital. In fact, the goals they have set are set with the patient's agreement. But one has to question how much, or how was the patient told how much she is likely to achieve. 'Do you think you would be able to.' Nine times out of ten the patient will conform, rather than saying, 'I don't think I can.' Cutting from say thirty cigarettes a day to say twenty a day, or no smoking at all. You are asking a lot of the patient.

e/a: It talks about being fairly successful about reducing Mrs Forest's weight. But reducing her smoking has been less successful. I think that should have been looked at in more detail. Probably by another discussion with the patient because she is a factory worker, she is not likely to be extremely stimulated. Maybe smoking eases her tension.

i: I suggest that other things related to health education should have been brought in there. Either to think of it in terms of self-help groups, relaxation or other methods. Possibly a little bit more about a healthier diet.

nd: I honestly think that there is a little bit of conformity going on here from the patient. Agreeing with what has been set out.

i: Maybe at that stage she is referred to somebody like the liaison health visitor. I would suggest that whilst she is still in hospital she should be referred to people who will be able to help her, say for example, the dietician. Mrs Forest being allowed to talk and discuss her own anxiety about her diet. If she has got a family, you don't know what the budget is like in the family, the financial situation, that may influence what they are eating at home.

e: Although people are mentioned here. I think there are a few assumptions. The patient is agreeing to everything. I would, as a sister, say that she is agreeing too easily.

p: I don't know if she will achieve all that has been set when she goes home, or even stick to it. We would probably need to give her a lot more support in relation to changing and trying to promote a healthier lifestyle.

i: I mean, it's nice to see she was referred. But she is actually referred to a health visitor for coronary patients. One could argue that you are labelling her. Although she has got ischaemic heart disease. Maybe you are trying to push the point too much, thinking of all the other aspects.

Vignette 7

l/pi/a: I think it stems around the fact that he is a forty-five-year-old school teacher, happily married with two teenage children and that no one in the family has suffered any serious illness with regards to him having diabetes. There is the fact that he is going to have it for the rest of his life and he is to have insulin for the rest of his life. Consequently, he is showing psychological problems relating to this; the effect it is going to have on him; the change in the lifestyle at home; coping with teenage children; how they are going to react to it as well. It seems sudden, because he has to give his own injections. That seems to be part of the problem. The fact that he has got diabetes and totally feels inadequate as a person. I think he views himself as a failure, rather than viewing it as something that could happen to anybody. He is going to have difficulty coming to terms with the fact that he has got this illness and that it is going to be with him for the rest of his life. But it doesn't mean that his life ends then, rather than just a few adjustments with his lifestyle. I think that he probably feels that his chances, career-wise and promotion, are not going to be there, because he is going to have an attack at school.

a: I would imagine that there needs to be a lot more discussion with the patient to allow him to expand on his feelings, regarding his loss of confidence and feeling inadequate. I think that it needs to be expanded on very much before we go on to take any action. There may be some of that which is a normal reaction, but there is an awful lot that isn't a normal reaction. I think that it is the type of lifestyle he leads that is going to cause an abnormal reaction to it.

i: Therefore, I think he needs a lot of counselling and support in the initial period.

pi: It is, I think, how he views himself as a person that is one of the problems.

Index